Weight Loss for Middle-aged Women:

7 essentials Fat Busting strategies to regain your ideal weight in 30 days

By Julie Clark

Table of Contents

Chapter 1:
The Best Weight Loss Workout Routine for Women

Okay, ladies, let's cut to the chase: each day of the week find the time to do the following workouts. No excuses. The sooner you want to get your ideal bikini body, the more intense your workout should be.

In all honesty, it does not matter which part of the day you should exercise right now. The most important rule is to simply do it everyday. The habit of regularly exercising will help get you in shape along with your healthy diet plan.

To help you create a specific workout plan that works for you, below are lists of important workout steps, details and options that you can choose from so that you can never grow bored with the same old routine.

Equipment

As a beginner, all you will need is a pair of 5-pound dumbbells, a basic yoga mat and a pair of running shoes.

You can keep using your dumbbells until they become weightless to you after weeks of training. After that, you can increase them to 8 pounds or you can increase the number of reps.

A mat is important for exercises that will require you to be on the floor or on your hands and knees. This will prevent injury, friction burn or pain in your bum whenever you do certain workouts.

Running, jogging and power walking are very basic yet highly enjoyable workouts that require a sturdy and comfortable pair of running shoes. Make sure to research on the best pair for your foot type, form and gait.

Warm up

There are plenty of warm up exercises out there, but here's a quick, 3 to 5 minute warm up set that you can do to start:

- Head rotation - clockwise and counterclockwise, 20 reps

- Forearm rotation - 30 reps inwards, 30 reps outwards

- Arm rotation - 20 reps inwards, 20 reps outwards

- Shoulders rotation - 10 reps inwards, 10 reps outwards

- Wrists rotation (hands together, fingers clasped) - 20 reps clockwise, 20 reps counterclockwise

- Torso swings - 15 reps per side

- Torso bends - 20 reps per side

- Hips rotation - 10 reps clockwise, 10 reps counter clockwise

- Knees rotation - 10 reps per leg

- Feet rotation - 10 reps per leg

- Scissors (abs warm up) - horizontal for 30 counts, vertical for 30 counts

- Reverse V (stomach on the ground, arms and legs pointing up to form a V) - 20 reps

Cardio Workout: three times a week

Cardio is extremely important for it strengthens the heart and lungs, lowers stress, encourages sound sleep and helps you burn calories fast. Aim for 20 to 30 minutes of intense cardio or 45 to 60 minutes of light cardio.

Here are some great suggestions on how to start your cardio workout:

At the gym: treadmill, rowing machine, stationary bike, stair stepper, arm ergometer, interval training, circuit training

Group classes: spinning, salsa dancing, Cross Fit, Zumba

Outdoors: jogging/running, cycling, power walking, swimming, rock climbing

At home: (best accompanied with an instructional video) dance aerobics, hip hop, cardio kickboxing, Tae Bo, jump rope, hula hoop

Strength Training: two to three times a week

Having stronger muscles will make life easier for you overall. Keep in mind that strong muscles is not equivalent to bulky muscles. Only a specific diet will trigger bulkiness if paired with strength training. Aim for at least 2 rounds of strength training each week to boost your metabolic rate and really enable you to drop off a lot of excess weight.

Reps and Sets: with each session, aim for 1 set of 12 to 15 reps (short for repetitions of one full move) with each exercise on the first three weeks. After that, aim for 2 sets with 30 to 60 seconds of rest in between sets.

Basic Strength Training for Weight Loss: There are tons of free strength training workout videos that you can find online and follow. Here is a list of the most important basic strength workouts that you can look up and follow based on target muscles:

- Biceps: Standing and seated dumbbell curls, dumbbell preacher curls

- Triceps: close grip push-ups, overhead dumbbell triceps extensions, laying dumbbell triceps extensions

- Shoulder: seated and standing overhead dumbbell press, dumbbell upright rows, dumbbell lateral raises and front raises

- Abs: abdominal crunches, prone planking, abdominal hold, side crunches, The Hundred, squat thrust with twist

- Back: dumbbell rows, dumbbell shrugs, pull-ups, chin-ups

- Quadriceps: dumbbell squats, front squats, split squats, lunges, step-ups

- Hamstrings: leg curls, dumbbell Romanian, Straight Leg and Sumo deadlifts

Flexibility Workout: two to four times a week

The amazing thing about flexibility training is that you can do it in between the seemingly "more intense" cardio and strength workouts because it leaves you feeling more relaxing and less strained. However, it still makes you break up a sweat, improves your performance in the other two workouts, and helps you lose weight as well.

Do at least 5 to 10 minutes of flexibility training. If you can, do it before a cardio or strength workout. Otherwise schedule it on days when just want to exercise lightly or when work keeps you really busy.

Here is a list of amazing flexibility workouts that you can look up online and include in your workout plan (hold each pose or stretch for 10 to 30 seconds):

- Basic Yoga poses

- Basic Pilates

- Upper body: Shoulder and Chest, Arms Across Chest, Triceps Stretches

- Lower body: Glute, Adductor, Single Leg Hamstring, Standing Quadriceps, Standing Calf Stretches

Cool down

At the end of each workout session, allow yourself at least 15 minutes to cool down before you hit the showers to avoid getting sick.

While there are plenty of cool down exercises out there, you can follow the basic upper and lower body flexibility exercises stated above as your way of cooling down. After that, do a simple Yoga pose called the "savasana" or the Corpse pose for total relaxation. Finally, enjoy your post-workout snack and a tall glass of detox water for another 5 or 10 minutes before you take a bath.

Recommended Weight Loss Workout Week Plan

Here's a very easy-to-follow daily workout guide that evenly spaced out intensity throughout your week. It's ideally made for women who have regular work weeks but if you have a different work schedule then you can always adjust the weekend workouts to your days off:

- Sunday- flexibility (light)

- Monday- cardio (moderate)

- Tuesday- strength (light/moderate)

- Wednesday- cardio (moderate)

- Thursday- flexibility (moderate/intense)

- Friday- cardio (moderate/intense)

- Saturday- strength (moderate/intense)

Each week, mix up the different types of exercises under each workout category and have fun!

Chapter 2:
The interconnection of Physiology and psychology- the special consideration of women psychology

The human body is a systematic orientation of various systems and biological patterns. The whole body functioning is based on an amalgamation of various bodily operations. Even the slightest change in the body's chemical and biological system can lead to serious malfunctioning. Nevertheless, this sensitivity is helpful in a way that it can give signals for even the slightest need for maintenance or check up.

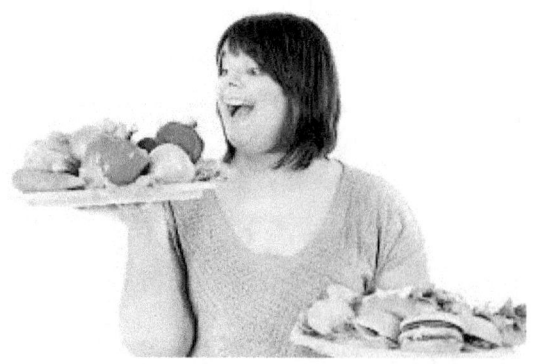

Although hundreds of ailments and body issues are in search of human health but if you talk about the most reported issue, obesity will surely come among the toppers in the list. The modern world has transformed the living patterns and eating habits altogether. The physical activity has almost diminished from the human life, as every activity has a substitute in the form of some technological invention. The Same transformation has occurred in the eating patterns. The natural dietary elements have been replaced by hundreds of artificial flavors and processed diet plans which have left obvious marks of obesity to people all around the planet.

Obesity has become a universal nightmare. Both men and women of all age categories are equally suffering from weight gain issues. So rather than straight away putting you into starvation techniques, it is better to understand the phenomenon more in-depth .Our main focus is the female group who struggle daily to maintain an average weight.

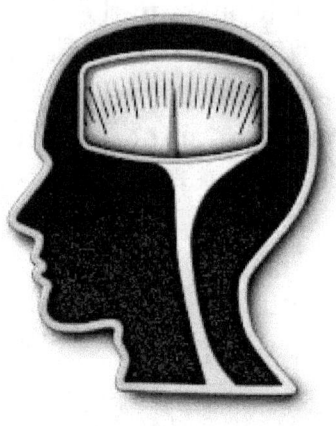

Weight gain is both physical and psychological:

The reason for writing this book is to divert the attention of people towards the psychological domain of obesity, which has been overlooked since so long. Everyone is running behind various diet plans and exercise in order to shed pounds. But the psychological connections have been overlooked for so long. It is now time to unveil the underlying connections between the two.

Whether one is slim or fat it is considered as a physical condition of the body but the psychological impressions are also connected with it. If one is not happy from the attire and overlook of his or her body, it can have a great effect on the overall psychology of the person. It can lead to disappointment and discontentment. This virtual cycle can go a long forever, in which the person being obese becomes restless and disappointed so much so that he refrains from any kind of effort to overcome this situation. Disappointment leading to no input to the issue leads to more weight gain and it becomes a self-fulfilling prophecy.

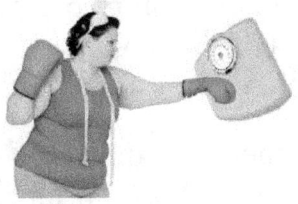

Women are more prone to psychological traps:

Women are known to be fragile creatures that possess various distinguishing psychical and psychological features. Experts are of the view that women get more affected by obesity because they lack the control and determination which is needed during the weight loss venture.

- Women are more emotional, unable to cherish emotional management for them.

- Women are more possessive about their outlook

- Women are more judgmental and compare themselves from unrealistic ideals.

- Women want appreciation and acceptance with social circles.

- The fear of losing prominence makes them feel disappointed.

Considering these important psychological aspects of women, it is important to handle the weight loss issue from a psychological aspect as well. This book is intended towards this aspect so that enough of emotional and psychological strength can be gathered thus leading towards effective weight loss. The proper diet and psychological interventions both can create miracles for any kind of weight loss issues. Diet plans followed without any include determination and psychological strength will never reveal benefit, so let us consider the important psychological hacks for making up the way for weight loss.

1. Focus on the X and Y factors

2. Learn the psychological and physical domains of weight loss

3. Apply a health- belief model

4. Apply self-determination theory to your weight loss venture

5. Dig up the meaning of "dieting"

6. Understand the barriers to being "slender"

7. Consider psychological deprivation cycle

8. Always remember about inaccurate comparisons

9. Focus on self-monitoring

10. Build up a strong support system

Chapter 3:
Apply the rules of psychology to get a "thinner" you

1. Focus on the X and Y factors

Based upon the traditional struggle which is put forward for weight loss by the majority of the victims around, you can write a simple formulaic presentation of this struggle. It will be:

Weight Shedding = Diet plan + workout

The majority of you will agree upon this. Almost all of us agree, so we try looking up the latest trends in diet plans so that we can get the best for the first part of input in the formula. Same is the case for the second part. The trendiest technology has made exercise a form of science, where every individual can get customized solution for a workout that can help him or her in gaining the optimum or ideal weight.

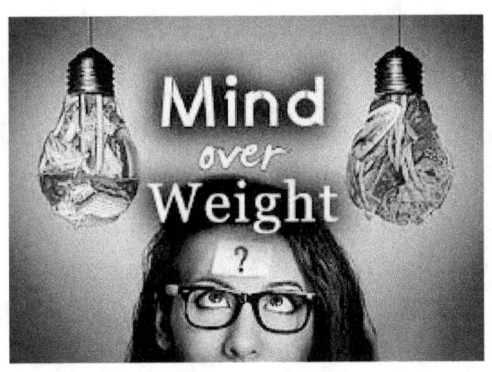

But this is an incomplete picture or ineffective illusion of the real picture. Weight loss is more than this, especially for women.

- **The corrected formula (implication of X and Y factors)**

Now if the above formula is incomplete, how can we make it correct so that the real struggle can result in obvious results. Obviously, the output side of the equation will stand still because the ultimate goal is to lose weight.

But from the input side, two significant and highly decisive factors are missing and always overlooked. Let us suppose these factors to be X and Y, such that:

Factor X = Adherence and devotion to the weight loss treatment

Factor Y = Personal change

With these factors added to the above formula, there will be no reason for a woman not to accomplish weight loss as it is the absence of these factors which makes the whole venture incomplete.

- **Adherence and devotion to the weight loss struggle**

Like any other venture or important campaign, weight loss is also a struggle. It is a fight within you, which leaves its results in the form of physical outlook and a number of pounds shown on a weight machine. But when you lack the devotion for this struggle, the diet plan and work put plans all are of no use.

Start with the basic questions and find the most realistic answers to these questions.

- Why do you want to be slim?

- What personal factors are involved in struggling for weight loss?

- What social factors are involved in struggling for weight loss?

When you will answer these questions you can easily categorize the motivational forces which can work for you. Out of these motivational forces, choose the one that can make you more devoted to the cause.

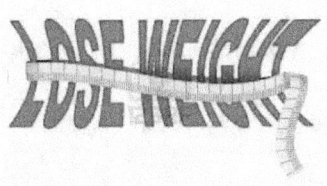

Women are known to be emotional, a bit more than men. It gives the vulnerability to get a victim of disappointment. But they need to make their selves realize that weight loss is not a game for a day or two. It is a long quest which can put up results only when followed with adherence and continuous efforts. If a woman possesses Devotion to continue fighting, she is already half the way nearer to her dream.

- **Personal change**

It is not all about starvation and keeping yourself restricted from the scrumptious and tasteful duets. Neither is it only about spending hours and hours on the treadmill. Weight loss requires a personal change. For that a woman needs to cater following important issues:

- What can motivate you?

- What is the biggest hurdle in your way of weight loss?

- What are top three reasons for failure?

- How do you learn about weight loss?

- Have you set specific goals for weight loss?

- Who are you as an individual with some specific sources of uniqueness?

- What your daily routine has to do with losing weight?

- How do you see your personality?

- What is the level of your defenses?

- What is the level of your openness?

- What is the level of your closed-mindedness?

- What is your personal history?

- What is the nature of your self-perception?

- What are the social comparisons which you make?

- What do you believe about your success in weight loss?

- What are the ways you pursue for monitoring yourself?

- What are the ways you pursue the feedback about weight loss results?

- What are the points of personal conflicts?

- What are your feelings regarding defeat in weight loss?

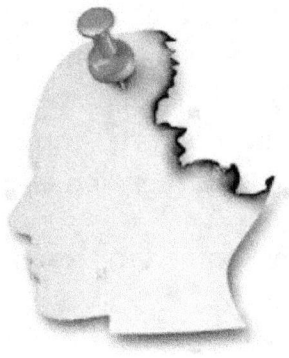

2. Learn Psychological and physical domains of weight loss

This is an extension of the corrected formula which was discussed earlier. The physical domain is related to all which you put in the form of physical struggle, like restricting yourself from eating and spending hours for physical effort. But a human body and human life cannot be fully catered if the psychological domain is left unattended. For that the psychological domain pertaining to weight loss will include following major aspects:

Self-control

Self-control is being capable of resisting the inner force which drives you against your struggle. Under self-control women will be able to cater the efforts which demand an exit out of their comfort zone so that they can put more than the standard effort. You will find clear usage of self-control when you are:

- Being determined to Exercise Self-Control

- Being accustomed to "Saying No"

- Being able to Resist temptation

- Having an Effortful control

- Resisting self-denial

- Being able to stay firm

- Putting off gratifying yourself

- Having power of mind

- Being committed to your long-term goals

- Keeping the focus high

These self-control abilities will allow you to make use of physical aspects of weight loss with a greater input. In this way, you will be able to g quicker and finer results. As women are believed to be emotional and quite delicate so they give up earlier as compared to men. So this psychological hack is especially useful for women.

Self-Appreciation

Most of the time the biggest reason for the ineffectiveness of weight loss struggle is the inability to notice the progress. Women are usually at a higher risk of getting trapped in this phenomenon. The lack of confidence makes them unaware of their hidden talents because of which they are unable to see up the performance. Sometimes there is not a large count of pounds which needs to be given off. Only a little appreciation can make her feel better. The inability to self-appreciate is the psychological reason why women do not feel satisfied with their weight loss. If exercise and diet plan is followed with a self-appreciation about the struggle, it will lead to a motivational cycle of putting a higher level of struggles. Eventually, the results will get better with every passing day. When you will start appreciating your outlook, the devastating effects of extra pounds, if any, will also lessen. This perfect match of physical and psychological effort will leave no space for any kind of ambiguity.

3. Use health- belief model

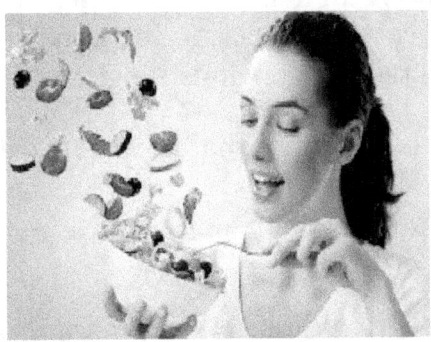

Health belief model is a psychological model which is based on the framework of expectancy-valence. Although it is an old model, yet it has been applied recently to the concept of obesity and weight loss. Under this model, two important phenomenon reside closer to the need of attention.

- Locus of control

- Self-efficacy

When this particular model is extended towards the weightless struggle, it narrates that one will feel motivated towards weight loss when:

a. He has a belief that losing weight will reduce their risk of getting a life-threatening sickness

b. He has an internal locus of control making him expect that his or her self-effort will direct specific behaviors which will result in obvious weight loss.

c. He is confident that he is able to carry out the behaviors and activities which are mandatory for weight loss.

These points clearly predict that valuing a particular outcome, which in this case is the attainment of ideal weight through weight loss activities, and believing one's self to be able to achieve that result uphold motivation.

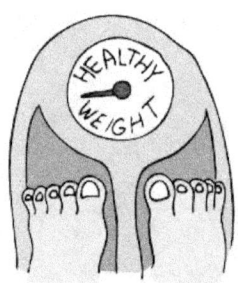

Here the critical point is to look up for various types of motivation

- **Autonomous motivation**

The famous self-determination theory of psychology states that autonomous behaviors are the ones for which the guideline is practiced as chosen and as appearing from one's self. Being connected to inner being of the individual autonomous motivation is related to the internal locus of control and causality also takes place from within

- **Controlled motivation**

Under the effect of controlled motivation, behaviors are said to be *controlled* behaviors for which the regulation is experienced as forced or pressured or by some external intra-psychic force or interpersonal factor. Hence, it is related to the external locus of control.

So applying these psychological principles to your weightless activity you will find new principles of successful weight loss. These principles related to the long-term maintenance of weight loss, which would *not* result from merely dieting if the reasons extended for dieting were purely controlling. So if a woman is going to gym only because his spouse wanted her to be slim and she feels guilty of not doing so, then her motivation for Weight lose activity is purely controlled. Here the external locus of control will come into play and that woman will not be able to endorse the behavior personally. The willingness to go to the gym will not be personal. Here the activity will be pursued as a burden and hence the result will also be limited.

On the flip side, if the motivation for the same activity would have come from within, then the same women would have pursued weight loss with more control and passion. This internal motivation can be developed by creating awareness about the health benefits associated with optimum weight or by having an internal desire to look young and fit. The same activity will yield fruitful results. So if you are not getting effective results, you need to look for these ways.

4. Apply self-determination theory

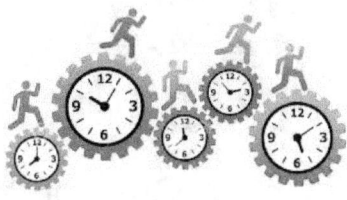

This is another important psychological domain which can be extended to the issue of weight loss which people are facing. This theory connotes that the regulation of a particular behavior of a person depends on upon

- Individual difference

- Social-context variables

In this case, the focus of attention is to see the behaviors and set of activities related to weight loss, this may include following specific diets and pursuing work out session.

Within the individual difference orientation which leads to regulation of behavior, the person will have three major concepts

- The autonomy
- The control
- Impersonal orientation

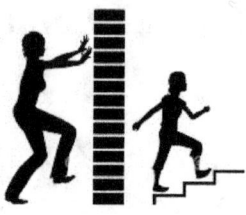

The autonomy perspective for weight loss complies that there is always a general ability to be self-regulating in losing weight and to learn the contextual factors that endorse individual choice and personal initiative.

Autonomy orientation applied to weight loss will also create other positive behaviors like self-actualization, integration of personality and self-esteem. In this case, all those contextual factors which relate to this inner motivation will be seen as a support mechanism and person can continue with weight loss activities. Whenever this autonomous perspective will loosen the grip, the chances of getting back are greatly enhanced.

Now self-determination applies that all those women who are not finding the positive or visible result of their weight loss activity, need to internalize their effort, whenever they will pursue dieting or exercise as a pressure, they will never be able to get the maximum behavior.

You may have seen people who have maintained their weight and exercising routine for the past so many years. It is because they had developed an internal passion for doing so, in earlier years of their struggle and now the waves of motivation come from within.

Stand in front of the mirror, look up yourself and put up a dialogue with your own self. Convince and motivate yourself about pursuing weight loss venture. Extend reasons and maintain and evaluative feedback loop.

Chapter 4:
Stand out of the "Usual"

5. Dig up the true meaning of "Dieting"

In a past survey, it was reported that almost 60% of Americans are either obese or gaining weight at a high rate. The Same survey reported that out of all dieting attempts, 90% end up to be a failure. These figures are of a society where there is a whole industry pertain to dieting products and exercise aids.

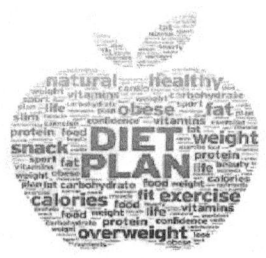

The word "dieting" is quite familiar to all of us, especially women. Women usually have a history of pursuing variable and trendiest "diets." They start it with a passion and motivation, follow the diet and shed off some initial pounds. With the passage of time, the downfall starts and motivation for dieting starts fading off. Women usually regain the lost weight at this stage and some may even gain more than the previous number of pounds. So the question arises about the ineffectiveness of these diets. But in reality, it is more of a psychological game.

If we relate the dieting perspective with the psychological issues of a person and especially of a woman, we will see following chief issues.

- **Unrealistic Expectations**

Apart from the inner mental model, it is somewhat related to untrue marketing campaigns, the diets usually claim unrealistic results and women buy and follow he diets with the expectation that the same results will be achieved. For example, the diet packages may claim that lose 10 pounds within 5 days and a woman starts believing that after these 5 days her life will be at ease.

- **Rigid Rules**

When a diet plan is too rigid to follow, it is hard to continue it with full motivation. Especially if a person had been into excessive eating, he or she will need extra will power to continue these diets with rigid rules.

- **Elimination of specific nutrients**

The market is full of fat-free, carbohydrate free or protein-free diets, so subtracting whole nutrient out of your life is really had to pursue.

- **Defining a Beginning and an End**

Women usually pursue dieting with some definite view. The common examples are, "I am going for a diet from this Monday." Dieting cannot be pursued with these definite markings.

6. Understand the barriers to "thinness"

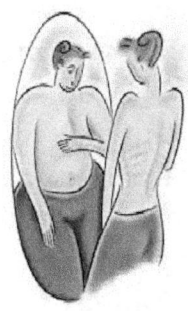

In this society, everyone wants to be the first one in the list. This over emphasis on the attainment of best possible has made us look for ultimate ideals. Same is the case with the ability to look good. We have started focusing on outlook so much that it has led to a never-ending struggle of looking good.

• The need to Redefine thinness:

There is a difference between being healthy and being lean. If you are underweight, look slim but your internal body systems are weak, it will surely lead towards a number of body issues. The top results will be a loss of immunity which can drag to a number of dangerous results. So there is a need to define and prioritize thinness.

- **Inability to see accurate self-image:**

Women are sometimes unable to self the accurate self-image. It is because of their insecurities and lack of confidence. Sometimes women are having a group of friends having an extra slim figure. This put them in a situation which blurs their accurate image. They cannot see their inner beauty and outer magnificence and tart struggling for the same figure; an accurate self-image can keep you away from the unneeded struggles.

- **Formulate a personal solution for thinness:**

When the above two steps of defining the thinness with reference to an accurate self-image will be completed, you can get into the step of forming a customized solution for weight loss. It will help you to stay away from the rule of thumb type diets and exercise plans. Most of the weight loss activities result in faded results because they have been designed with a general perception about obesity and weight gain. Customized solutions always yield better results.

7. Psychological deprivation cycle

It is an important psychological hack which can make you understand the real cause of your failure for not being able to get desired results.

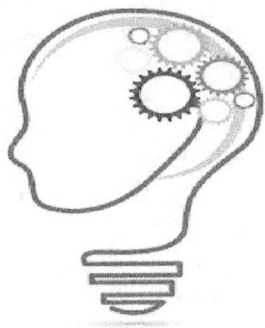

- **Rules:**

The first thing which is followed din case of diet or exercise is to set up "rules". These are like the judgmental phrases, depicting the goodness or badness of a particular behavior.

- **Breaking the rules**

Under the effect of these rules, the person will see certain food as either good or bad. For example under your diet rule brownies were bad for weight loss. Now you were on a get together hand your find has served you the brownies. What will you do? Most probably you will eat. It is also because you were a lover of brownies.

- **Psychological deprivation:**

Although you will eat brownies but your mind will keep on signaling that you have broken the rule. It will send disappointment signals to the brain and you will feel low about your weight loss struggle. Eventually, there will be no motivation left.

It is better to cherish your mind with loss connections rather than getting into hard and fast rules.

Chapter 5:
Nothing Stands Impossible

8. Always remember about inaccurate comparisons

One of the biggest mistakes which lead women to suffer from unsuccessful weight loss venture is the tendency to indulge in inaccurate comparisons, under the influence of these incorrect comparisons women tend to feel discontented and discouraged.

- **Illusions about ideals**

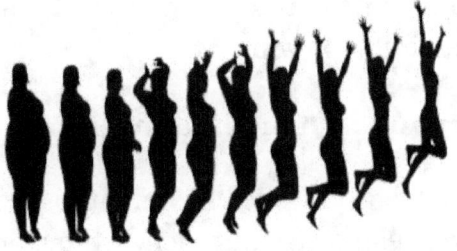

We being suspected to illusions, sometimes see the outer shell of any entity. Women see models, actors, and fellows who have unusually slim bodies. But we never know, from what they are suffering from. Unusual leanness may be the result of some hidden disease or it may have been a gift of genes. So women just start the struggle for reaching the ideals with a false illusion of their perfection. Get rid of this false illusion about ideals or you may render never ending disappointment

• **Refigure the ideal**

As far as weight loss is concerned, women are mostly concerned with weight loss because of their possessiveness to beauty, outlook and a slim figure. However, it is just an incomplete view. A healthier and accurately working body is much more needed. If you weigh lesser than your age, it can be a signal of some hidden disease. In order to achieve successful weight loss, it is necessary to compare your performance with the most optimum solution which can have long-lasting benefits for you.

• **Everyone is "One in a million"**

One of the biggest issues in weight loss of women is their relative approach, they need to understand their uniqueness and their individuality, without which success is not possible, and this uniqueness needs to be considered at every step, from crafting diet plan to making an exercise routine. Even the ideal weight cannot be same for two persons. So sometimes which a woman is labeling as unsuccessful weight loss may be a successful one, under the specific contextual and surrounding factors.

9. Focus on self-monitoring

This is the biggest hack which can reveal miracles. No one can make you follow the path of weight loss, except yourself. Under the influence of self-monitoring you can achieve a number of useful benefits.

- If you had been into compulsive or Binging or eating, only self-monitoring can stop you. Eventually, the results start to appear as more obvious and clear. Compulsive eating is usually done without restriction so the self-restriction can act as a moderator for this relationship.

- Self-monitoring will also keep you away from Overeating till it diminishes away fully.

- Under the self-monitoring effect, the psychological deprivation cycle will get slower as you will not feel an external check on your activities. There will be "A No Rule" policy" which will make you feel more satisfied with the results.

- Under self-monitoring excessive eating will get diminished and eventually the extra pounds will be lost sooner. Sam will be the case of going to exercise or gym.

When ideal weight will be achieved self-monitoring can help you to maintain this weight throughout because maintenance is also a motivational task.

10. Build the Strongest Support System

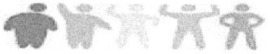

Throughout this book, we have mentioned that losing weight is surely challenging. It is quite a long way to go. Throughout this venture, there come unlimited challenges and hardships which make a person to go on the back foot. All psychological aspects discussed above were related to individual personality but this last hack is from a social perspective. We all need to support each other for making up healthier society

- **Generate positive energy**

Try to get in touch with the strongest support system, the members of this support system can be your friends or your colleagues or your family members. But the eventual purpose of this support system is to make you continue your struggles. This support system extends positive energy which is needed during weight loss. Weight loss is usually accompanied by lack of confidence and determination but positive energy can enhance the strength.

- **Constant motivation**

When constant energy is dissipated, the eventual result is motivation. women usually lack the motivation, although they may be following the ideal diet plans and exercise routine but with a lack of motivation, they feel disappointed and unsuccessful. Under the effect of motivation, any weight loss venture can turn out to be a real miracle.

Chapter 6:
Increasing Your Chance of Success

In order to ensure your success with my weight loss program, I have listed several strategies that will help you stay on track and get through those early days. But please remember, they will only work for you if you follow through with my suggestions.

Because you will be on your own, it is important to know how to identify, and therefore avoid, the common obstacles and pitfalls that could disrupt your progress.

To guarantee the effectiveness of my tactics, I've also had my wife incorporate them into her own weight loss journey. The response from her was more than good. Several of her friends also asked her for guidance after seeing how well she managed to lose weight and then maintain it.

Time and again I've given these strategies to friends and family to try, so I know they can be invaluable. This is especially the case for those of you who are working your way through this weight loss plan alone.

Please don't be tempted to jump over this next chapter. I strongly recommend you invest some time reading it carefully. What comes next can really do wonders for your overall motivation, and therefore see you successfully lose three pounds in a week!

Handling Lack of Motivation

So, you have now made a conscious decision and decided to start your life anew. This may or may not be the first time that you have chosen to lose weight and improve your overall health, but I can promise you this: Stick with the program and you WILL achieve your goals, and for that you need to know how to fend off signs of demotivation.

Staying focused and motivated is something all of us are challenged with from time to time. Motivation is that psychological feature which keeps us going, and helps us to stay enthusiastic about working towards a specific target. Without it, none of us would be able to accomplish our weight loss goals.

The question here is how do you avoid, or get rid of, any negative thinking that creeps in? When my wife wanted to lose weight she asked me for my best motivational tip, and the one that would make her get through those days when she just wanted to lie on the couch, or throw in the towel altogether.

I think she was hoping to hear something quite spectacular, and was evidently disappointed by my response. I simply said to her: *"Just do it, no matter what, even if there is a tornado outside."* Alright, so that's a bit extreme, but she got the gist of what I was trying to say.

In my experience, the biggest mistake people make with regards to health and fitness is thinking that someone else will do this for them, or some magic shortcut will be handed down. Personal trainers are great for keeping the motivation up, but most of us can't afford, or justify the cost, of hiring one.

Blocking Negative Thoughts

A simple way to maintain your motivation levels, particularly during longer periods, is to use something that I simply call 'blocking negative thoughts'. This basically involves disallowing yourself to feel down, thus avoiding the trap of demotivation.

One example of how this might work in practice is to stand on the weighing scales and realize that you are not even close to your goal. In this case it's easy to lose motivation and think *"Oh what the heck, I will never lose weight, so what's the point of trying?"*

However, if you are able switch your thinking pattern from the negative to the positive (by forcing yourself to think different thoughts if you have to), then you will be able to block these destructive feelings.

Just tell yourself to keep working towards your goal no matter what. Tell yourself that you CAN do it, and the results you will get in the long term are going to be truly amazing, trust me on this. You CAN do it!

In my experience, this approach is usually what separates the people who are able to lose a significant amount of weight from the ones who spend their whole life trying. The first group is able to grip their teeth and workout even when it's the last thing they want to do, whereas the second group succumbs to the temptation of quitting!

Although this mindset of 'just do it' is easier said than done, there are other techniques you can adopt to get your motivation back, or even build on the motivation you already have.

I am personally using these methods in my daily exercising, and to be honest, I would have a hard time accomplishing what I do without them.

These techniques are discussed in the following chapters and will really help you to stay focused and motivated. I strongly recommend that you to read them and look at ways to include these into your routine as well. You will get the best results out most of your weight loss journey if you do.

Stay on the Right Path

When it comes to successful weight loss, nothing is as important as staying on the right path. Even when you experience setbacks for whatever reason, or relapse into old habits, you need to know how to quickly pick yourself up and get back on track.

It's too easy to throw in the towel and convince yourself that you can't do it anymore, or I that you will try again some other time. This old frame of mind has no place in your new approach for achieving those goals, and so it has to go.

I'm assuming your main objective is to lose weight, which is why you are reading this book. And I'm also going to assume that you are serious about this because you have already read down this far.

Having said that, deciding to lose weight is one thing, but actually doing it is something else. So I urge you to invest some time into learning how to get through failures and setbacks during your journey, because they will transpire occasionally; they always do!

Having patience, persistence, and a strong determination to succeed are the attributes that will steer you clear from failure. Providing that you take heed of the things you learn in this book, then working towards your goal, and keeping on the right path, will be so much easier.

An example of getting off the right path is to imagine yourself eating something you shouldn't, like a brownie or a chocolate bar. In this case you have just abandoned the right path and allowed your mind to move over to old ways of thinking.

Okay, so it's only a thought, but it is this kind of pondering that will eventually take you onto the wrong path, and potentially lead you into acting on the temptation. Just remember, all actions start with a thought!

Whenever these thoughts come into your head (usually quite uninvited), you need to kick them out immediately and not allow them to linger. The only way to do this is to replace the bad thought with a good one; something more positive and goal orientated.

There's no shame in failing once, or even a few times on your journey to lose weight. Most successful outcomes have had some failures or setbacks along the way, but the point is to get back on track and not look at these letdowns as permanent stumbling blocks.

I say again, the important thing here is to immediately move back onto the right path and don't let the disappointment keep you down. Or as Fred Astaire and Ginger Rogers remind us in that famous duo of theirs, you simply pick yourself up, dust yourself down, and start all over again!

The key thing here is learn to accept your failures and realize that they are a natural part of your weight loss journey. Just accept them and take them for what they are, without too much reflection.

Losing weight is not a lesson in torture, so don't beat yourself up, just keep pushing forwards and you will quickly take back control, of that I can promise.

If you think about it, what can you do if you have eaten that brownie or skipped a workout? I mean, you can't turn back the clock, but you can stop reflecting on your mistakes and move on.

After all, it's impossible to move forward if you're always looking back, so there's no point in harboring regrets.

When my wife first tried to lose weight, she sometimes stumbled off the right path and gave into temptations. Occasionally she would make the mistake of eating something she shouldn't, or just skip a workout and spend the time lounging in front of the TV, giving lame excuses for her procrastination.

Once the setback had occurred, she would call me and say how bad she felt about doing this, or not doing that. But I always encouraged her and said that there is absolutely nothing to worry about by these mistakes, so long as she learned something from them, and got back onto the right path again.

Immediately she would feel better and sound much happier, realizing that it's not the end of the world. If you don't have someone who can encourage you, and give you a little inspirational push when you most need it, then form the habit of encouraging yourself instead.

This kind of self-encouragement usually works best when you speak the words out loud, and not merely try to think your way into a better frame of mind.

When it comes to losing weight, it is you who needs to persist through any failures and setbacks and keep yourself on the right track. No one else can do it for you. It's really important to remember that!

Chapter 7:
The First Seven Days

This is a very simple plan that I have been using for years to help my friends and relatives lose weight. I have modified it a bit to suit your 7-day goal, and also adapted a few things so that anyone can follow it regardless of their age.

It is different to all the other fast weight loss plans out there because of the food selected. I've turned this plan into a mini-guide for clarity. It's all about staying as simple and as straightforward as possible, while at the same time allowing for a little diversity!

Each day has its own specific plan outlined that you need to follow in order to achieve the desired results. Do not cheat or modify your meals in any way, if you do, then there is a real risk that you will not get what is expected, which is that 3 pounds weight loss over a seven days period.

OK, so, if your chief aim then is to lose three pounds in a single week, you need to know that this equates to about 10,500 calories.

To give you an idea of how much you are expected to burn, I will list some popular foods that you are not allowed to consume during this plan.

The 10,500 calories you are supposed to burn over the coming week is equal to seven regular-sized pizzas. While this may seem like a huge number, I can assure you that if you follow my plan of action without cheating, you will easily accomplish this!

Day 1

The first day is the toughest, if for no other reason than the sudden change in diet will be a bit of a shock to your body.

How much of a shock depends on the individual, and the foods they are accustomed to eating. Now, unless you are clinically obese then you should be able to get through day #1 without too much fuss.

I am not saying that it's going to be plain sailing, but you need to really focus on achieving this goal without cheating. Remember, what you get out of it depends on what you put into it.

Exercise

Your exercise for today is to walk at fair pace for 10 km (6.2 miles). I consider the 10 km distance something you should be able to get done if you just focus on the task. And try to enjoy it because it will make the walk so much easier.

Although the distance might look massive (especially if walking any distance is alien to you), please be mindful of the fact you are getting something in return for your effort.

This may not be a picnic, but at the same time it's not a lesson in torture either. Your goal is to lose weight, and that's going to take a little effort. However, never lose focus on why you're doing this, and things become so much easier, I promise.

Breakfast

- Oatmeal with maple syrup (1 cup)

- Orange Juice (1 cup)

- Turkey Bacon (3 slices)

- Big glass of water (zero calories!)

Snack

- 1 apple

Lunch

- 2 turkey sandwiches, on whole wheat bread with ¼ cup of cheese & mustard

- Big glass of water (zero calories!)

Snack

- 1 apple

Dinner

- Mixed greens salad with ¼ cup of cheese

- 4 ounces of cooked salmon (filets work great here!)

- Big glass of water (zero calories!)

Summary

This day was all about getting the working week off to a great start. There's a foundational breakfast, a quick lunch, and a dinner that you should have found quite satisfying.

You also walked 10 km (6.2 miles), which is just fantastic, and you should be proud of yourself. Don't forget that when it comes to exercise, it gets easier over time, not harder, so don't worry if you feel a little stiff and worn out on day one because that's perfectly normal if you're not used to it.

Day 2

If you are reading here, then you're ready for day two, so well done you. Now, if you stuck to Monday's plan, Tuesday will help you stay the course.

You will find avocado to curb off hunger pangs, along with a healthy mix of fruit that will help you stay lean and avoid refined sugars. Remember that drinking water is a zero calorie activity, but you can also enjoy coffee and tea without sugar.

Exercise

When you woke up this morning, did you feel a few minor aches and pains as a result of the long walk yesterday? My guess is you did (unless you're used to exercising), otherwise you must have taken some shortcuts (remember, no modifications to this plan).

Today, I have a surprise for you. I need you to walk again, only this time a little bit further than yesterday. The target distance is 11 km (6.8 miles)!

I know it sucks, but 'no pain no gain', right! Let me just reiterate what I said earlier: exercise gets easier over time, not harder, and once you get past these early hurdles, there's a good chance that physical training will get into your blood, and become something you want to do, as opposed to something you feel you need to do, and then you will thank me.

Remember that earlier on in the book you agreed to abide by the rules when committing to my weight loss plan. This means you have no excuses for not fulfilling your duties.

If you are aching after yesterday's exercise, try to get a short massage before today's walk if you're in a position to do so, as it will help increase your blood flow and decrease the hurting somewhat.

Breakfast

- Breakfast shake of blueberries and bananas blended together with 2% fat milk and 1 tablespoon of honey

- Big glass of water (zero calories!)

Snack

- 1 apple

Lunch

- Tortilla filled with half an avocado, 2 hard-boiled eggs (chopped up), with mustard

- Big glass of water (zero calories!)

Snack

- 1 apple

Dinner

- Half an avocado (saved from lunch)

- 1 large chicken breast

- Mixed salad greens

- Balsamic vinegar for salad

- Big glass of water (zero calories!)

Summary

This day is probably the one that decides whether you will continue with my weight loss plan of action or throw in the towel. However, I am hoping will not give up, and are ready to face day three.

Try never to lose sight of why you are doing this, and keep your mind focused on how you will look and feel by following through to the end.

Day 3

OK, so here we are at the middle of the week – how are you doing so far? I've decided to keep things a little lighter on today's menu, even though your workout routine will be slightly tougher!

Exercise

Welcome to day three. If you've made it this far, you are doing just great, so keep pushing forward. Today I have put your walking exercise back to 10 km (6.2 miles), but you are also required to perform the following exercises too, in order to pass the day three goal:

- 15 sit-ups (3 sets), rest 1 minute in between

- 10 pushups (3 sets), rest 2 minutes in between

This is something that you should be able to get through with a little bit of sweat and effort. I know it's a pain to do these types of exercises, but I promise you they are necessary, and they won't take long.

Tip: You can do the pushups by resting on the knees instead of your toes, if that helps. That said, I do suggest you to try performing them on your toes if you can, because it's more efficient that way.

Breakfast

- 1 bagel

- 1 cup of yogurt

- Big glass of water (zero calories!)

Snack

- 1 pear

Lunch

- 2 turkey sandwiches with ¼ cup of cheese and mustard

- Big glass of water (zero calories!)

Snack

- 1 apple

Dinner

- 1 baked white potato

- ¼ cup of cheese

- 1 cup of tomato soup

- Big glass of water (zero calories!)

Summary

You've just completed the third day and you really should be very proud of what you have achieved so far. I know that your feet are probably hurting, and you feel like you've been hit by a train.

Don't worry though, this is how it should be as both your mind and body adjusts to doing things outside of your comfort zone.

Don't you dare give up now that you've come this far! Remember, what I said earlier, 'no pain no gain', so keep looking forward and remember why you're putting yourself through this.

Tomorrow is a new day with new challenges, so get some well-earned rest to recharge your batteries, and prepare yourself for day four.

Day 4

Almost done! You should be feeling great by now; at least I hope you are! Usually when I work with friends and relatives on this course of action, day four is when they start feeling better and more enthusiastic.

We're going to get back into the meal plan today, with a tasty treat at the end: a nice healthy portion of ribeye steak. Mmmm... delicious!

Exercise

Today's goal is a little bit different because I want you to vary your walking speeds for 10 km (6.2 miles). I know it may feel like quite a hike at this distance, but it is necessary if you're to lose the expected weight.

What I want you to do is walk at the highest possible pace you can for 1 km (a little over half a mile), and without stopping.

I suggest you do this after the halfway mark. This will give your body ample time to be properly warmed-up, and therefore increase your chances of making it. Try not to quit as you feel lactic acid (burning sensation) build up in your legs. Instead keep pushing forward knowing that each step is closer to the end. Don't forget to remind yourself why you are doing this. Stay focused and I'm sure you will make it.

Breakfast

- 2 fried eggs

- 1 cup of oatmeal

- 16 fl oz of coffee (for your travel mug)

- Big glass of water (zero calories!)

Snack

- 1 apple

Lunch

- 2 tuna sandwiches (toasted)

- Big glass of water (zero calories!)

Snack

- 1 pear

Dinner

- 4 ounces of ribeye with 1 pat of butter

- 1 cup of mushrooms

- ½ cup of onions

- Big glass of water (zero calories!)

Summary

So, how did it go? Did you manage to walk at the higher pace for 1 km (little over half a mile), and without stopping? If you didn't, don't worry, it's not that a big deal. What's most important here is that you tried, and you still did the 10 km.

The idea of walking at a higher pace is to involve a little bit of what's known as 'interval training' in your walking. What this does is help to speed up your metabolism slightly, and that's just great for burning off more fat!

Tomorrow is a whole new day, and it's going to be a bit tougher yet again. Make sure you prepare yourself well by resting this evening and getting a good night's sleep. Remember not to diverge from the nutritional recommendations given either (very important!).

Day 5

Hooray! You're almost done – for real! The weekend awaits you, but today is all about feeling full, changing things around a bit, and trying out new things.

Exercise

Because you've come this far, you can't give up now, no way, not on the goal line. Instead you need to keep pushing forward, even if it's the last thing in the world you feel like doing!

So, what have I prepared for you today? Well, you are still supposed to walk the 10 km (6.2 miles) as usual, but you should also try to add a second interval into it.

After walking for about 4 km, you should walk at high pace for 1 km (little over half a mile). Then walk for another 4 km and then again at high pace for 1 km.

As you can see, I have added one more interval to your walking routine, and yes, it might be a bit painful, but I am sure you will be able to make it now that your body is adjusting to the exercise. Good luck.

Breakfast

- ½ cup cottage cheese

- 1 cup of oatmeal

- 4 slices of turkey bacon

- Big glass of water (zero calories!)

Snack

- 1 apple

Lunch

- 2/3rd cup of tuna salad mixed with egg

- Big glass of water (zero calories!)

Snack

- 1 pear

Dinner

- 1 cup of rice pilaf

- 3 cups of mixed salad greens

- 2 tablespoons of Caesar salad dressing (low calorie)

- 4 ounces of chicken breast

- Big glass of water (zero calories!)

Summary

Today you are at day five of my seven-day weight loss challenge, and almost at the end, so don't you dare give up now! You've been doing absolutely great so far, but hey, you don't need me to tell you that!

Now, make sure to rest this evening and get a good night's sleep. Once again, follow the nutrition plan above or you could undo all that hard work if you stray from the course. Tomorrow is a brand new day filled with new challenges!

Day 6

Just because it's the weekend, that doesn't mean you have to 'fall off the wagon', or succumb to temptation. You can continue to eat well, lose weight, and feel even better with each passing day, Saturday included!

Exercise

I must say, I am truly proud of you now because you've come so far in my program. Okay, so you are probably wondering what I have prepared for you today, especially with regards to the workout. Well, don't worry, there is no huge difference as it's going to be similar to the one you did yesterday, albeit with a little extra added!

I have included the strength training from day two, and also increased the number of reps slightly! Besides walking for 10 km (6.2 miles) you are expected to accomplish the following exercises:

- 20 sit-ups (3 sets), rest 1 minute in between

- 12 pushups (3 sets), rest 2 minutes in between

Breakfast

- 2 pancakes with margarine

- 1 cup of milk

- 1 cup of blueberries

- Big glass of water (zero calories!)

Snack

- 1 apple

Lunch

- Tuna salad with chips

- Big glass of water (zero calories!)

Snack

- 1 pear

Dinner

- 4 ounces of roast beef

- 1 cup of mixed vegetables

- Big glass of water (zero calories!)

Summary

We're almost done now with just one day left to complete the seven-day weight loss plan. It must feel great to have come so far, right?

By now you should have a solid knowledge about nutrition and training, and know what you need to do to achieve successful weight loss.

As always, make sure to rest this evening and get a good night's sleep. Remember to stay on the path and follow the guidelines on nutrition as outlined above.

Day 7

Hurrah! It's the last day of the Quick-Start program. You should be feeling fabulous, and even seeing some changes in the mirror after just one week of following my plan. Less bloated? Feeling lighter? It's all part of the strategy.

Okay, so you might have had to reduce meal portions (quite a bit for some of you), but that was obviously done on purpose.

A lot of people overlook how much food they're actually eating, and it's a well-known fact that the vast majority of us eat far more than we actually need anyway.

Give it time, stick with your new lifestyle, and you will naturally start to feel fuller on less food: that's a given.

Exercise

I hope that you prepared for today and raring to go? I bet you are because today is the last day of the program, and needless to say it's also going to be the toughest.

But you are almost done now, so there's no point of even thinking about giving up! Furthermore, you will be in better shape on day seven than you were on day one, so even with the extra exercise, today will still most likely seem easier than that first day.

Now, today I have increased the challenge a bit by changing your routine slightly. Yes, you are still going to cover the 10 km (6.2 miles), but this time you should try walking at the higher pace for at least one third of the distance. Here is the plan:

- Walk 2 km, and then walk at a higher pace for 1 km (little over half a mile)

- Walk 3 km, and then walk at a higher pace for 1 km

- Walk 2 km, and then walk at the higher pace for 1 km

I am confident that you will make it through this last challenge and keep pushing forward. Don't forget, your finish line is just around the corner now.

Breakfast

- 16 ounces of coffee (enough for 2 cups)

- Smoothie of blueberries and bananas in milk (1cupof blueberries, 1 raw banana)

- Big glass of water (zero calories!)

Snack

- 1 cup of yogurt with 1 tablespoon of honey

Lunch

- Whole wheat tortilla stuffed with 2 hard-boiled eggs (chopped up) with tuna and low calorie Caesar dressing

- Big glass of water (zero calories!)

Snack

- 1 apple

Dinner

- 1 cup of cooked shrimps

- 1 cup of tomato soup

- Big glass of water (zero calories!)

Summary

If you have followed my nutrition and workout instructions exactly as I wrote them, then you should have lost an average of 1,400 calories each day!

The Result

At the beginning of this book you learned that an average women needs to be under 2,200 calories per day in order to lose weight. You have consumed 1,400 calories per day which gives you a minus of 800 calories.

However, you have also burned 700 calories each day by exercising. This now gives you a total amount of minus 1,500 calories per day (equal to 300g of chocolate).

This gives us a total of 10,500 calories which is equal to three pounds of your weight (3,500 calories per pound).

An easy way to control this is to check your weight in the morning. Make sure that your water intake is normal the previous day, and don't eat before weighing yourself.

If you find that you have not lost three pounds in weight, then you need to go back and see where you have gone wrong. Hopefully, you have been keeping a journal, which will make it easy to go back and figure out where you went wrong as you compare each of your days to the ones outlined in my weight loss plan.

Maybe there was a day where you could not resist junk food, or perhaps you were unable to control the size of your plate (check the rules of the plan for details).

Whatever you find out, you should correct it and repeat the seven-day challenge (which will be much easier the second time around).

You should only continue reading further if you have achieved the three-pound weight loss goal. If not, you need to go back and repeat it for as long as necessary in order to reach the objective.

Only then will you be ready to take that achievement further, and develop it to fit in with your new, happier, healthier, and slimmer lifestyle.

I also recommend you reread the chapter on 'Handling Lack of Motivation', and let it sink in because it's really important.

The only person responsible for your weight loss is yourself, and not anyone or anything around you. Remember not to beat yourself up if you failed to reach the target goal.

The important thing is that you tried and will continue to try. The saying I often like to quote here is: "The only real failure in life is the failure to try."

Please understand that all I have done here is to give you the tools required to reach the goal. Whether you accomplish that goal or not is down to you.

Chapter 8:
The Next 7 Day Weight Loss Meal Plan – Way to Lose 20 Quick Pounds

If you believe that you are good to start following this meal plan to burn down body fats, there are some things which you must be aware of. The first and most imperative aspect's to get yourself mentally prepared for the dietary regime you are about to pursue. It is very significant to have a peaceful and controlled mind in order to acquire all the possible benefits which are offered by this quickest method of losing weight. This whole meal plan will be executed in seven days. All through this time you will have to strictly intake only those foods which are prescribed in it for each day of this week. If followed in the way this meal plan is mentioned, it's believed that you'll reduce around 20 pounds.

One more thing, those who are planning to follow this 7 day weight loss meal plan must know that losing weight quickly is not about starving at all. In point of fact, keeping yourself hungry and skipping meals could do the exact opposite and you may end up pulling in some extra pounds. This superb weight loss meal plan is especially designed and it suggests the ideal amount of foodstuff that you could consume, which will keep you always satiated.

Some people may be curious and thinking about how a weight loss meal plan could be effective if it is allowing its followers to eat certain foods. In addition to it, those folks who relied on this seven meal plan were mystified about how a weight loss program doesn't ask its pursuers to fast and will aid in effective and quick weight loss. However, in reality, there's nothing to be worried about when taking up this weight loss plan, since it's an absolutely sure shot process which is carefully designed by the experts to diminish your weight by 20 pounds in a matter of 7 days. So, buckle up yourself and get started with the day one.

Day 8 Fresh Fruits All The Way

Most of the folks are well aware of this fact that the day one of any venture is considered as the most imperative time, and this battle of weight loss is no exception. It is the moment when you are getting yourself prepared to step into the arena of knowing every secret of losing excessive body fats in merely in the time span of 7 days. This quick weight loss meal plan suggests that on the very first day you must significantly rely upon the fresh fruits along with some other low-calorie foods. The best thing about it is that you are allowed to eat just about all kinds of fruits that you love. However, it is imperative to stay away from bananas. This restriction is particularly for the first day only. Cantaloupe and watermelons are some highly recommended foods that one could consume.

The followers of this weight loss meal plan should also consume loads of waters (around eight to twelve glasses) on the day make. In addition to it, it is extremely crucial to ensure that you steer clear of any food item which offers a high amount of calories, even from the boiled or raw veggies. If you are really looking forward to make this weight loss plan does its work efficiently then you ought to eat as much fruit as you could on the day one all through this day. In case, you still feel hungry, then do not panic and eat your other favorite fresh fruits and obviously consume water.

Day 9 Veggie Can Be Very Nutritious

If the first day of this fastest weight loss meal plan provided you the chance to binge upon all of your favorite, fresh and juicy fruits, then the second day is going to give you an amazing opportunity to consume just veggies all through the day. The followers of this diet plan are allowed to eat all those vegetables they like both in cooked and raw form. However, it is extremely vital to ensure that you never use any kind of cooking oil in order to cook your veggies. Eating a decent amount of boiled veggies is a great option as well. You can boil any vegetable you might want to, including potatoes. Although, it will be much safer and better if you choose to eat potatoes in the earlier part of the morning. This way, your body will be able to burn down carbohydrates throughout the remaining part of the day.

Boiled cabbage, cooked beans, lettuce, cooked and raw carrots, ridge gourd and boiled bottle, cucumber and broccoli are some of those veggies which are particularly recommended to consume on the second day of this weight loss meal plan. Without a doubt your digestion system will undergo a complete renovation by the second day's evening. That is why; you would have to hit the washroom quite frequently than before. Aside from eating tons of vegetables, it is also imperative to make certain that you don't forget to consume your dose of eight to twelve water glasses on the day two.

Day 10 Fruits and Veggie Combo

On the third day, you will be allowed to consume both fresh fruits and veggies for the whole day. But, you must ensure that on this particular day you stay a thousand miles away from one constituent of the fruits section that is bananas and also ensure you don't intake an ingredient from of the vegetable section that is potatoes. Potatoes must not be taken in any form, neither boiled nor grilled. On the third day of this weight loss meal plan, you can go for a vegetable diet in early morning, which is followed by an appetizing fresh fruit diet for the midday and a veggie dieting in the late afternoon and once again fruit diet before you go to bed.

The good thing about this amazing weight loss meal plan is that it is quite flexible and the biggest example of its flexibility is that on the third day you have the option as well as the combinations and permutations of eating the veggie and fruit diet or the blend of both of them is left totally up to the followers disposal. In other words, it is up to you to settle on whatever you will love to eat provided its vegetables and fruits. Do not miss the vital element of today's diet plan which is the consumption of eight to twelve pure water glasses.

Day 11 Banana Filled Day

The fourth day will interest those dieters who want to get rid of more or less twenty pounds in a mere seven days, since it's crammed with a milk and banana diet. You will have to eat at least eight to ten bananas all through this day and could consume up to three milk glasses. Some people may be a little anxious if this suggested meal plan will make them feel hungry. However, in reality, all followers will feel hundred percent satiated throughout the day. Meanwhile, you will have to break up the consumption of the milk glasses and bananas in a proper way in order to avoid starvation on day four of this 7 days quick weight loss meal plan.

Taking a milk glass and a banana in the earlier part of the morning, which is followed by two bananas in the afternoon, will be the perfect beginning of the fourth day. You can consume 3 bananas and a milk glass in the late afternoon, and finally the last glass of fat free milk and three to four bananas at night. If the plan is followed in the right way, there would be no indication of starvation at any moment of the day.

Day 12 Juicy Tomatoes

Those who love to relish feast will find the fifth day of this fastest weight loss meal plan the most interesting, since it allows all followers to have a buffet on day 5. On this day one could have a medium sized cup of scrumptious rice at lunch and can consume around 6 to 7 fresh tomatoes all through the day. Since there will be a great chance of generating loads of acid that is why it is strictly advised to amplify the overall consumption of water from twelve glasses to fifteen glasses on the fifth day.

Day 13 Water and Veggie Mix

It is virtually not impossible for you to find the fastest weight loss meal plan which lets you feast twice in the whole week. Just like fifth day, here too, followers of this diet plan are allowed to consume a medium sized bowl of rice at lunch and for the remaining part of this day they can rely upon a veggie diet. The water consumption on the sixth day must be maintained in between eight to twelve glasses. As it is the penult day of this quick weight loss meal plan, then you must feel pretty much lighter than you were before six days. There is nothing to be doubtful about that you'll be completely enhancing your digestive operations as well by taking up this 7-day meal plan.

Day 15 Fruit Juices

It is the final day of your 2nd phase weight loss meal plan. On this day you can consume some vegetables along with a cup (medium sized) of rice. It is also recommended to drink some fruit juices as well, but it is vital to ensure that you only consume 100% natural and fresh juices. The processed and packaged juices are a definite "No no". It is probably the best and ripest day of this whole meal plan since you can consume any veggies of your preference

Chapter 9:
Breakfast, Lunch and Dinner Plan in the 3rd Phase Days Weight Loss Meal Plan

During this week of struggle to get rid of 20 pounds, one can also follow the following diet on each day of this amazing 7-day weight loss meal plan.

Day 16

Breakfast: Flossy Pancakes

- Combine one and a half cup of yogurt (low-fat), in a medium sized bowl along with ¾ cup of milk (fat free), one cup of pancake mix of buckwheat or whole wheat and one egg.

- This scrumptious recipe makes around five servings. You can eat one now and the four individual servings can be packed away in the fridge for forthcoming meals.

- It can be served with two tbsp of maple syrup, fresh strawberries (one cup) and one cup milk (fat free).

Lunch: Egyptian pea Salad

- Get a medium sized bowl in order to combine canned Egyptian chickpeas, one and a half tsp white vinegar, ¼ tsp black pepper (ground), one tbsp black olives (sliced), ¼ cup of green pepper (chopped), ¼ cup of white onion (chopped) and two tsp olive oil.

- Mix all the ingredients thoroughly and serve the dish over two cups of lettuce leaves.

Dinner: Healthy Chicken kebabs

- Slice four ounces of a chicken breast (raw) into small sized chunks, so that they can be easily put on a kebab stick.

- The small chunks of chicken breast should be marinated for at least thirty minutes in the Italian dressing (¼ cup fat-free).

- Slice green pepper and white onion into chunks and set out ten grape tomatoes.

- Swap cherry tomatoes, pepper, onion and marinated pieces of chicken chunks on grill and skewers.

- It can be served with a pita pocket of whole wheat, which must be browned on the grill.

- Spread the pita pocket with two tbsp hummus. Finalize it by one cup of milk (fat-free) mixed comprehensively with one tbsp of strawberry mix.

- In order to relish added refreshment, you can freeze the luscious strawberry mild right into a mold of Popsicle. Enjoy this healthy dessert with the lip smacking chicken kebabs.

Day 17

Breakfast: Yogurt Cold Cereal Parfait

- Take a glass and layer six ounces of fruit flavored light yogurt with two tbsp granola (low fat) and one cup of raspberries.

- Start with the third part of yogurt, third part of raspberries as well as third part of cold cereal.

- Continue mixing till each and every ingredient is well layered.

Lunch: Veggie Pot Pie

- Start heating one Swanson's Chicken or Amy's veggie pot pie by following the directions given on the package.

- Serve with ten grape tomatoes.

Dinner: Mozzarella and Tomato Sandwich

- Finely slice baguette roll of six inches in the half lengthways.

- Sprinkle shredded mozzarella (thirty three percent reduced-fat) on the halves of baguette rolls and put it in the oven toaster for around four to five minutes at the temperature of 250 degrees, till cheese's just starting to melt down.

- In the meantime, slice two red large tomatoes. Once done, take out the baguette from oven and sprinkle some dried oregano and dried basil on it if desired.

- For the topping, you can put some slices of tomatoes over baked baguette.

Day 18

Breakfast: Goat Cheese and Chive Frittata

- Preheat oven to three hundred and seventy five degrees Fahrenheit. Take a medium sized bowl with a fork and mix pepper, salt, milk and eggs. Stir in chopped chives and diced tomatoes.

- In a nonstick skillet, melt butter on medium temperature.

- Pour in the goat cheese right on the egg mixture's top. Cook for three to four minutes.

- Put skilled in an oven and bake for nine to ten minutes. Enjoy!

Lunch: Artichoke & Turkey Sandwich

- Spread two medium sized slices of the bread with one tbsp of light mayo.

- Stuff the slices of bread with three ounces of sliced breast of turkey, 1/3 cup of shredded mozzarella cheese (reduced-fat) and four to six artichoke hearts.

- Serve with one cup of red or green grapes and fifteen baby carrots.

Dinner: Chicken Scaloppine on Broccoli Rabe

- Take a medium sized skilled and heat some oil in it over high temperature.

- Mix pepper and breadcrumbs in a dish and dredge the pieces of chicken in the mixture of breadcrumbs.

- Put chicken in a frying pan. Cook each side for three minutes. Once done, take it off from the pan and keep warm.

- Add butter, juice and broth in a pan. Put in the broccoli rabe and cook for three minutes.

- Now add capers and parsley in it.

- Serve the chicken over the mixture of broccoli rabe. Garnish with the slices of lemon. Keep the leftover for tomorrow's lunch.

Day 19

Breakfast: Fresh Raspberries and Fluffy Pancakes

- From the Monday's breakfast, sever some delicious fluffy pancakes with one and a half cup of fresh raspberries, two tbsp maple syrup and one cup of milk (fat-free).

Lunch: Chicken Scaloppine on Broccoli Rabe

- Serve the remaining chicken scaloppinie on broccoli rabe from the Wednesday's dinner.

Dinner: Baklava and Frittata

- Get the remaining chive frittata which you made for the Wednesday's breakfast and serve it with two cups of leaves of the baby spinach, which can be topped with one cup of milk (fat-free) and two tbsp balsamic vinegar.

- Have one slice of toast (whole wheat) and top it with two tbsp of margarine (fat free).

- For dessert, get a two inch baklava piece, which is a famous Greek pastry.

Day 20

Breakfast: Crunchy & Creamy Yogurt

- Serve six ounces of light yogurt of any flavor you like in a medium sized bowl which should be topped with one cup of cereal (high fiber).

- You are allowed to select one hundred calories of just about any of your favorite cereal like a half cup of the Raisin Bran or one cup of cherries. Top with the three tbsp of crushed walnuts.

Lunch: Veggie Pita Sandwich along with the Greek Cucumber Sauce

- Mix a half cup of plain yogurt with a half chopped cucumber, half clove of garlic (minced) and a pinch of pepper and salt, if preferred.

- Spread half quantity of the yogurt (put aside the leftover for later on utilization) on one pita.

- Fill pita with one cup of string beans and five chopped grape tomatoes.

- Serve with one cup of fresh cherries.

Dinner: Broccoli Rabe along with Soy and Sesame

- Take a large sized saucepan and boil eight cups of pure water in it. In the boiling water, cook broccoli for two minutes. Once done, drain.

- On medium temperature, heat a nonstick skillet of large size. Add some peanut oil it and whirl it in order to coat.

- Now add garlic and crushed pepper in the pan and cook for thirty seconds, while stirring occasionally.

- Put broccoli rabe in a pan and cook for two minutes. Add black pepper and salt.

- Gently toss the sautéed broccoli rabe in sesame oil, sugar, rice vinegar and soy sauce. Enjoy this healthy recipe!

Day 21

Breakfast: Creamy Peanut Butter over Chocolate and Bagel

- On a bagel (whole wheat) of one ounce, spread one tbsp of peanut butter.

- Serve it with one cup of milk (fat free) mixed with two tsp of chocolate syrup as well as one cup of green or red grapes.

Lunch: Lip-smacking Pizza with Salad

- Have one large slice of cheese pizza with thin crust (choose veggie toppings like onions, peppers or mushrooms) along with two cups of green salad topped with two tbsp of any regular dressing.

Dinner: Lamb Souvlaki with Rice at Your Preferred Greek Restaurant

- At the second last day of this 7-day weight loss meal plan, you deserve to have some dining at your favorite Greek restaurant. However, you still have to order only those cuisines which are healthy, yet have low amount of calories so that you can keep your weight off and get yourself prepared for the next round of the 7-day weight loss meal plan.

- At eatery you can order a lamb souvlaki. You can have lamb of a soup-bar-size amount along with rice of the baseball-size quantity. Go on and eat up all veggies that you get with this order. If some part of the order remains, then you can get it packed for the Sunday's lunch.

Day 23

Breakfast: Pita Along with Raisins and Ricotta Spread

- Take a pita (whole wheat) and fill it with a 1/3 cup of ricotta cheese (fat free) and mix it with one tbsp each of honey and peanut butter.

- Sprinkle one tbsp raisins right on the mixture of pita. Enjoy!

Lunch: Lamb Souvlaki with Rice

- Eat the leftover lamb souvlaki with rice from the Sunday's dinner.

- You can serve it with one cup of cooked spinach or two cups of baby spinach.

Dinner: Summer Salad - Basil Shrimp

- Marinate nine large sized or twelve medium sized shrimps in a marinade of basil for thirty minutes.

- In order to prepare basil marinade, mix ¼ cup of white vinegar, 1 tsp of dried basil or 1/8 cup of fresh chopped basil, one tbsp lemon juice and one tsp olive oil.

- Grill your shrimps till they are cooked through.

- For added flavor, top two cups of the romaine lettuce along with the shrimps.

- Serve with one cup of fresh berries.

Day 24:

Breakfast recipes:

Buckwheat and Quinoa Granola

Ingredients

- 3 tbsp. of honey

- 3 tbsp. of liquid coconut oil

- 1 tsp. of vanilla extract

- ¼ tsp. of ground cinnamon

- ¼ tsp. of ground ginger

- 1 cup of buckwheat oats

- 1 cup of cooked quinoa

- ½ cup of old-fashioned oats

- ½ cup of unsweetened cranberries (dried)

Preparations

1. Prepare oven with a 325°F temp.

2. Prepare a baking sheet with light grease, or ready your silicon baking mat.

3. Mix your honey, coconut oil, vanilla extract, cinnamon, and ground ginger in a small bowl.

4. Set aside first.

5. Then, mix buckwheat, quinoa, and oats in a large bowl.

6. Blend in your honey mixture thoroughly.

7. In prepared pan, spread the mixture evenly to be baked evenly as well.

8. Bake it in your oven preheated to 325°F.

9. When grains start to brown, usually takes 40 to 45 minutes, remove and mix in cranberries.

10. Make sure to cool it completely before placing in airtight storage.

Cherry Quinoa Porridge

Ingredients

- 1 cup of water

- 1/2 cup of dry quinoa

- 1/2 cup of dried unsweetened cherries

- 1/2 tsp. vanilla extract

- 1/4 tsp. ground cinnamon

- 1 tbsp. honey (optional)

Preparations

1. Stir all ingredients except honey in a medium-sized saucepan.

2. Over medium heat, bring it to a boil

3. Gradual stirring to avoid burning.

4. Lower the heat.

5. Cover and simmer for 15 minutes.

6. Done when quinoa is tender and all the water is absorbed.

7. Put in cup and drizzle with honey.

8. Enjoy your healthy breakfast.

Gingerbread Oatmeal

Ingredients

- 1 cup of water

- ½ cup of old-fashioned oats

- ¼ cup unsweetened cherries/cranberries (dried)

- 1 tsp of ground ginger

- ½ tsp of ground cinnamon

- ¼ tsp of ground nutmeg

- 1 tbsp. of flax seeds

- 1 tbsp. of molasses

Preparations

1. 1.In a small saucepan, mix all water, oats, cranberries or cherries, cinnamon, and nutmeg.

2. 2.Turn heat on medium-high.

3. 3.Bring the mix to a boil.

4. 4.Reduce heat and let it simmer.

5. 5.Let the water be reduced or slightly absorbed, usually it takes 5 minutes.

6. 6.Mix in flaxseeds.

7. 7.Let it stand for about 5 minutes, covered.

8. 8.Drizzled it with molasses and served.

Gluten Free Strawberry Crepes

Ingredients

- 6 cups of strawberries (sliced)

- 2 tbsp. of sugar or honey

- 4 large eggs

- 1 cup of unsweetened almond milk

- 2 tbsp. of light olive oil

- 1 tsp. of vanilla extract

- 1 tbsp. of light brown sugar

- ⅛ tsp. of salt

- ¾ cup gluten free flour (baking mix)

Preparations

1. Mix your strawberries and sugar in a clean container.

2. Let it stand for 30 minutes at a room temperature.

3. Whisk in eggs, milk, olive oil, vanilla, sugar, light sugar, and salt in a medium-size bowl until well-combined.

4. Blend in the flour and mix it well.

5. Heat a non-stick crepe pan, about 8 to 9 inch in diameter.

6. Pour about ¼ cup of the batter into the pan.

7. Swirl and to completely coat the non-stick pan.

8. Flip your crepe when it starts to turn brown to cook the other side. This usually takes 30 to 40 seconds.

9. The other side usually takes 10 seconds.

10. Be watchful to avoid burnt crepes.

11. Place it on a serving plate.

12. Spoon an about ½ cup of the strawberry mix and place it in the middle of the crepe.

13. Fold the crepe into a semicircle to cover the strawberries.

14. Drizzle the juices from your strawberry mixture for more flavors.

15. Serve and enjoy.

Raspberry Green Tea Smoothie

Ingredients

- 1½ cups of chilled green tea

- 2 cups of unsweetened raspberries (frozen)

- 1 banana

- 1 tbsp. of honey

- ¼ cup of protein powder

Preparations

1. With your blender, put in all the ingredients and blend.

2. Place in your favorite cup and enjoy.

Ginger Apple Muffins

Ingredients

- 2 cups of all-purpose flour

- ⅔ cup of sugar or sugar-substitute granules

- 1 tbsp. of baking powder

- ½ tsp. of salt

- 1 tsp. ground cinnamon

- 1 tsp. of ground ginger

- ¾ cup of unsweetened almond milk

- 1 cup of shredded apple

- ½ cup of ripe and mashed banana

- 1 tbsp. of apple cider vinegar

- ½ cup of crystallized ginger (finely chopped)

Preparations

1. Prepare your oven by preheating it on 400°F.

2. You can use paper liners, or if you are using a muffin pan, grease it lightly.

3. In a medium-sized bowl, blend in together flour, sugar, baking powder, salt, cinnamon and ginger.

4. Set aside and mix milk, apple, banana, and vinegar in a large bowl

5. Then mix in the flour mixture until blended well.

6. Fill your muffin cups in just about ⅔ full.

7. Start baking for about 15 to 20 minutes

8. Insert toothpick in the center, if it comes out clean, then you're done.

9. Serve with your favorite juice and have a healthy day.

Lunch Recipes

Boiled Fowl with Rice

Ingredients:

- ½ lb. rice
- A fowl suitable for boiling
- Salt and pepper
- 1 egg
- Butter
- Grated cheese

Preparation steps:

1. Cut up the fowl and boil until it is tender.
2. Wash the rice and blanch it by letting it come to a boil and cook a few minutes in salted water.
3. Finish cooking it in the broth from the boiled fowl.
4. Do not cook it too long or it will be mushy.
5. Add the broth a little at a time to be sure the rice is not too wet when it is done.

6. Season with cheese and butter and add the egg yolk to bind it just as it is taken from the fire.

7. Serve as a border around the fowl.

Spaghetti With Anchovies

Ingredients:

- ¾ lb. spaghetti

- 5 medium sized anchovies

- Olive oil

- Canned tomatoes

Preparation steps:

1. Put the anchovies into a colander and dip quickly into boiling water to loosen the skins, and remove the salt.

2. Skin and bone them.

3. Chop them and put over the fire in a sauce-pan with a generous quantity of oil and some pepper.

4. Do not let them boil, but when they are hot add two tablespoons of butter and three or four tablespoons of concentrated tomato juice made by cooking down canned tomatoes and rubbing through a sieve. Boil the spaghetti in water that is only slightly salted and take care not to let it become too soft.

5. Drain thoroughly and put it into the hot dish in which it is to be served.

6. Pour the sauce over the spaghetti, and if you have left the latter unbroken in the Italian style mix by lifting the spaghetti with two silver forks until sauce has gone all through it. Serve with grated cheese.

Vegetable Soup

Ingredients:

- 400 grams of mixed vegetables

- 200 g of pearl barley

- 1/2 onion

- 100 g of bacon

- 1 liters of vegetable broth

- 1 teaspoon of baking

- Oil of salt

- 1 package of croutons

Preparation steps:

1. Put the vegetables and barley to soak for at least 4 hours in warm water in the bowl of vegetables by adding a teaspoon of baking soda. Then rinse under running water, drain and set aside.

2. Cut the onion and powdered bacon into cubes and sauté with a little olive oil in a thick-bottomed saucepan.

3. Add the beans rinsed and drained completely of water and toast for a few minutes then add the farro (A type of hulled wheat, especially spelt or emmer, typically used in salads, soups, and side dishes).

4. Mix everything together then add the vegetable broth to completely cover the vegetables.

5. Put a lid and cook the vegetable soup over medium heat for about 40 minutes, stirring occasionally and adding more broth as you need it.

6. Remove the lid, add salt and pepper and cook a few more minutes.

7. Put on the bottom of each plate of toast, then pour the soup of barley and legumes.

8. Add some toast and then bring to the table your steaming soup of the house.

Spinach with Salmon

Ingredients

- 1 (5-ounce) salmon fillet, cooked

- 1 cup spinach leaves

- ½ cup red grapes

- ¼ cup shredded carrots

- 1 tablespoon sliced almonds

- 1 tablespoon dried cranberries

Combine ingredients in a bowl and enjoy.

Dinner Recipes

Farfalle with Mushrooms and Peas

This is a simple and delicious weeknight pasta. Serve this dish with whole wheat rolls and additional peas on the side.

Ingredients:

- 1 package (16 ounces) farfalle or other pasta

- 2 tablespoons olive oil

- 1 teaspoon chopped garlic (about 2 cloves)

- 2 pounds assorted sliced mushrooms (such as shiitakes, buttons, or criminis)

- 1 teaspoon fresh or dried thyme

- ½ cup chicken or vegetable broth ½ cup frozen peas

- ½ teaspoon kosher salt or ¼ teaspoon table salt

- ½ cup grated Parmesan cheese, plus additional for serving

Preparation:

Heat the water to cook the pasta according to the package directions.

Meanwhile, in a large skillet, heat the oil over medium heat. Add the garlic, mushrooms, and thyme and sauté them for 1 minute. Add the broth and simmer the mixture over medium-low heat, stirring it occasionally.

When you add the pasta to the boiling water. Add the peas and salt to the mushroom mixture. Cook the pasta until it is al dente.

When the pasta is cooked, drain it briefly, allowing some water to cling to the noodles, and return it to the warm pot over low heat. Add the mushroom-pea mixture and the Parmesan cheese and stir everything together until it is heated through.

Serve the farfalle immediately, topped with additional Parmesan cheese.

picking up speed Preparation times for the recipes are estimates, based on my experience making the dishes. If you are overseeing homework, stooping to scoop up blocks, answering the phone, or just taking your time (rather than Scrambling!), they may take you a little longer. I've noticed that recipes usually take longer the first time, so if a recipe becomes a family favorite, it may go more quickly.

Chicken Rochambeau

Ingredients

- 4 chicken breasts

- 4 thick slices of toast

- 4 thick slices of ham

- 4 glasses of red wine

- 1 pot of bearnease sauce

- 1 big handful of chopped parsley

- Salt & pepper

- 1 lemon

Prepare

Simmer the lemon, bay leaf, parsley salt and pepper in two inches of wine for ten minutes before adding the chicken to gently poach until cooked.

Artichoke Stew

Ingredients:

- 2 small lemons, halved, plus juice to garnish

- 15 baby artichokes

- 1/4 cup extra virgin olive oil

- 1 red onion, thinly sliced

- 1 teaspoon hot red pepper flakes

- 1/2 cup dry white wine

- 1 pound fresh peas, shelled

- 4 bunches scallions, root ends trimmed and whites and greens cut into 2-inch pieces

- Salt, to taste

- Freshly ground pepper, to taste

- 1 bunch fresh mint leaves

Directions:

1. Fill a large bowl with water and squeeze the lemon halves into it.

2. Remove and discard the tough outer leaves of the artichokes and trim the stems. Then cut the artichokes in half and scoop out the choke. As you work, submerge the halved artichokes in the lemon water.

3. In a Dutch oven, heat the olive oil over medium heat until hot, add the onion and cook until soft and translucent, about 4 minutes. Add the red pepper flakes, the wine, 1 cup of hot water, the peas, and the drained artichokes.

4. Cover and cook until the artichokes are just tender, 10–12 minutes. Add the scallions, cover, and reduce the heat to a simmer. Cook until the scallions are wilted and soft, about 4 minutes. Season with salt and black pepper.

5. Tear the mint leaves into pieces and sprinkle them over the stew. Garnish with a drizzle of olive oil and lemon juice. Serve warm or at room temperature.

Mushroom Stroganoff

Ingredients:

- 1 large yellow onion, chopped

- 8 ounces wild mushrooms, sliced

- 8 ounces white mushrooms, sliced

- 4 cloves garlic, minced

- 4 tablespoons whole wheat flour

- 3 tablespoons balsamic vinegar

- 1/2 cup soy milk

- 1 teaspoon thyme

- 16 ounces cooked fettuccini

Preparation:

Heat a non-stick skillet over high heat. Cook onions for 3 minutes.

Add mushrooms and garlic. Cook until mushrooms begin to release their juices. Sprinkle in the flour.

Stir until the flour is mixed in well. Add the vinegar and soy milk, stirring continuously until sauce is thickened.

Add thyme.

Serve sauce warm over cooked noodles.

Day 25:

Breakfast recipes

Eggs All' Aurora

Ingredients:

- 1 tablespoon butter or vegetable oil

- 1 cup milk

- 1 tablespoon flour

- 3 eggs

- Salt and pepper

Preparation steps:

1. Hard boil the eggs.

2. Make a white sauce of the flour, milk and butter. Be sure to cook it thoroughly.

3. Add the whites of the eggs diced very fine.

4. Pour this out on a platter and cover with the yolks forced through a sieve or potato ricer.

Corn Meal Loaf

Ingredients:

- Yellow cornmeal

- Dried mushrooms

- Parmesan cheese

- Butter

- Cream

- Salt

Preparation steps:

1. The day before this dish is to be served, cook cornmeal very thoroughly with only enough water to make it very stiff. Turn out to cool in just the shape of the dish in which it has cooked.

2. Next day take this same dish, butter it and sprinkle with bread crumbs. Cut the mould of cornmeal in horizontal slices about ¼ inch thick. Lay the top slice in the bottom of the dish where it fits.

3. Dot with two or three small pieces of butter and three or four dried mushrooms which have had boiling water poured over them and soaked some time. Moisten with cream and sprinkle with grated Parmesan cheese.

4. Repeat slice by slice until the shape is complete. On the last slice put only two dots of butter.

Put in a moderate oven and bake three hours. If at the end of this time there should be too much liquid on top pour this off to use for the seasoning of some other dish, such as spaghetti, rice or noodles, and continue cooking until the liquid ceases to ooze.

Breakfast Burrito

Ingredients:

- 2 lavash wraps
- 4 whole eggs
- 2 bunches of spinach
- 1 tomato, diced
- 1 cup sliced mushrooms cut
- 1 clove garlic
- salt
- Peppers
- Coconut oil or oil of your choice.

Preparation:

In a bowl mix 4 eggs, salt and pepper. Mix well with a wire whisk. While most will whisk you fluffier egg.

In a skillet cook the garlic, spinach, mushroom and tomato with coconut oil.

In a nonstick skillet cook the previously beaten egg.

Then place the filling in lavash wrap on and roll. Secure the roll with a toothpick.

Pancakes

Ingredients:

- 2 1/2 cups of flour (all-purpose)

- 2 1/2 cups of water

- 4 tablespoons of sugar (granulated)

- 2 tablespoons of canola oil

- 4 teaspoons of baking powder

- 1 teaspoon of salt

Preparation steps:

1. In a large bowl add the 2 1/2 cups of all-purpose flour, 4 tablespoons of granulated sugar, 4 teaspoons of baking powder and 1 teaspoon of salt and mix.

2. Slowly add the 2 1/2 cups of water and 2 tablespoons of canola oil and barely stir to mix. The lumpy mixture is to be expected.

3. Heat a large frying pan or griddle with a small bit of canola oil on medium high head.

4. Ladle the batter onto the hot griddle or pan and allow sitting until the edges become dry and bubbles form toward the middle.

5. Gently turn them over to brown the other side. Serve warm with drizzled maple syrup.

Lunch Recipes

Shrimp, Potato and Corn Chowder

Ingredients:

- 1 onion, chopped

- 1 bell pepper, chopped

- 2 carrots, chopped small

- 2 potatoes, chopped

- 2 16-oz bags of frozen corn

- 4 cups of chicken broth

- 1-pound shrimp, cleaned and peeled

- ½ cup heavy cream

- 1 cup water

- 2 tablespoons dried parsley

- 1 bay leaf, salt and pepper water and chicken broth.

Stir to combine. Cover the crock pot and cook on low for 6 hours.

Using an immersion blender, puree for 3-4 minutes, leaving it chunky.

Stir in the shrimp and cook for an additional 10 minutes.

When shrimp are cooked, stir in cream and salt and pepper to taste.

Sprinkle with parsley and serve.

Dinner Recipes

Brown Rice Stew

Preparation time: 15 minutes: Cooking time: 30 min max

Servings: 4

Ingredients

- 1 cup of brown rice
- 1/2 cup of walnut paste
- 1/2 cup of cashew paste
- 1/2 cup of almond paste
- 2 cup of coconut milk
- 1 tablespoon of palm oil
- A handful of fresh coriander
- 4 onions, diced
- 2 red chilies
- Salt and pepper to taste
- 1 tablespoon of cumin

Directions

1. In a pressure cooker, fry the rice and onions

2. Stir in the mushroom, and the chilies

3. Pour in the milk

4. Season with salt and pepper

5. Cover and cook for about 30 min

6. Release the pressure and serve hot

Slow Cooker Beef Fajitas

Ingredients:

- 1 ½ lbs. boneless flank steak, fat trimmed
- 2 large bell peppers, sliced
- 1 large yellow onion, sliced
- 1 (14-ounce) can stew tomatoes
- 1 ½ teaspoons chili powder
- 1 teaspoon ground cumin
- ½ teaspoon garlic powder
- ½ teaspoon salt
- Warmed flour tortillas
- Fresh salsa
- Fresh guacamole
- Shredded lettuce

Instructions:

1. Slice the steak into thin strips.

2. Combine the steak, bell pepper, and onion in a slow cooker.

3. Stir in the tomatoes, chili powder, cumin, garlic powder, and salt.

4. Stir until well combined then cover the slow cooker.

5. Cook on low heat for 8 to 10 hours or on high heat for 4 to 5 hours until the meat is cooked through.

6. Serve the fajita mixture on warmed tortillas.

7. Top with salsa, guacamole, and shredded lettuce, if desired.

Day 26:

Breakfast recipes

Mayonnaise, Egg and Bacon Potato

Ingredients:

- 750 grams potatoes (1 ½ pounds)

- 250 grams Mayonnaise (1 cup)

- 1-2 shallots, or 1 medium onion

- 6 eggs

- 5 rashers of bacon, chopped

- A small handful of chopped parsley

- Vinegar

- Sugar

- Salt and pepper

Preparation:

- Bring a small pan with water to boiling point, put the eggs in and boil for 10 minutes. Take out the eggs immediately and place in bowl with ice water.

- When cold, take off the shells, and cube the eggs. Finely dice the onion.

- Boil the potatoes: Place potatoes in a pan and cover with water. Cover with the lid and place on heat.

- Bring to boiling point, reduce heat, and boil until tender.

- Drain the potatoes, and let them steam off for about 10 to 15 minutes, or until cool enough to handle.

- Bacon: Place a little oil in a skillet on medium high heat.

- Fry the chopped bacon.

- Assemble the salad: Cut the potatoes into cubes of about 1 cm (1/2 inch).

- Mix the mayo, vinegar, onion and sugar. Mix in the potatoes, eggs, bacon and almost all of the chopped parsley.

- Season with a little salt and pepper.

- Mix, and sprinkle the remaining parsley on top. Place salad in refrigerator for a few hours.

Wholewheat Waffles

Ingredients

- 2 cups Spelt flour
- 4 teaspoons Baking powder
- 2 large Eggs, beaten
- 1 ¾ cups Milk, 2%
- 1/4 cup Sugar, raw
- 1 teaspoon Salt
- 1/4 teaspoon Cinnamon, ground

Directions

1. Preheat waffle iron to medium heat.

2. In a large bowl, mix flour, baking powder, eggs, milk, sugar, salt, and cinnamon.

3. Pour the mixture into the waffle iron.

4. Bake until done on both sides.

Breakfast Stack

Ingredients

- 6 ounces Potatoes, sliced

- 3 slices Canadian bacon

- 2 cups Spinach, chopped

- 1 large Egg, beaten

- 2 large Eggs, white only, beaten

- 2 ounces Cream cheese, fat free

- 4 slices Cheddar cheese, low fat, shredded

Directions

1. Preheat oven to 350 degrees F.

2. Layer in cupcake pan, sliced potato, bacon, spinach, egg mix and cream cheese, top with shredded cheese.

3. Then, layer another slice of bacon, egg mix, another slice of potato.

4. Bake for30-35 minutes and serve.

Lunch Recipes

Hearty Chicken and Vegetable Soup

You'll think this soup simmered all day, but it takes only thirty minutes to prepare. Refrigerate leftovers in the fridge for up to three days or in the freezer for up to a month so you'll always have some on hand for a quick meal.

- 1 teaspoon extra-virgin olive oil

- 1 medium yellow onion, diced

- 1 large carrot, peeled and diced

- 1 celery stalk, peeled and diced

- 2 (6-ounce) boneless, skinless chicken breasts, cut into 1-inch pieces

- 1 medium zucchini, diced

- 2 yellow squash, diced

- 1/2 cup chopped fresh parsley, plus extra for garnish

- 1 teaspoon chopped fresh oregano

- 1 teaspoon chopped fresh basil

- 1/2 teaspoon salt

- 1/4 teaspoon freshly ground black pepper

- 2 cups chicken stock

In a large, heavy skillet, heat the olive oil over medium-high heat. Add the onion, carrot, and celery and sauté, stirring frequently, for 5 minutes. Add the chicken and continue to sauté for another 10 minutes, stirring often.

Add the zucchini and squash, then the parsley, oregano, basil, salt, and pepper.

Sauté for 5 minutes, reduce the heat to medium, and pour in the stock. Cover and cook for an additional 10 minutes.

To serve, ladle into bowls and garnish with additional parsley.

Serves 2.

Mussels with White Wine

Mussels simmered in white wine is a traditional dish served all over the Mediterranean. It's ready in minutes, very impressive, and cannot be beat for pure comfort when served with crusty bread for sopping the juices.

- 4 pounds fresh, live mussels

- 2 cups dry white wine

- 1/2 teaspoon sea salt

- 6 garlic cloves, minced

- 4 teaspoons diced shallot

- 1/2 cup chopped fresh parsley, divided

- 4 tablespoons extra-virgin olive oil

- Juice of 1/2 lemon

In a large colander, scrub and rinse the mussels under cold water. Discard any mussels that do not close when tapped. Use a paring knife to remove the beard from each mussel.

In a large stockpot over medium-high heat, bring the wine, salt, garlic, shallots, and 1/4 cup of the parsley to a steady simmer.

Add the mussels, cover, and simmer just until all of the mussels open, 5 to 7 minutes. Do not overcook.

Using a slotted spoon, divide the mussels among 4 large, shallow bowls.

Add the olive oil and lemon juice to the pot, stir, and pour the broth over the mussels. Garnish each serving with 1 tablespoon of the remaining fresh parsley and serve with a crusty, wholegrain baguette.

Serves 4.

Dinner Recipes

Beef and Bean Chili

Servings: 4

Ingredients:

- 1 (15.5-ounce) can black beans, rinsed and drained
- 1 (15.5-ounce) can red kidney beans, rinsed and drained
- 2 (14.5-ounce) cans diced tomatoes
- 1 (12-ounce) bottle beer
- 1 lbs. boneless beef chuck, chopped
- 1 large yellow onion, diced
- 1 teaspoon minced garlic
- 2 tablespoons tomato paste
- 2 tablespoons chili powder
- Pinch cayenne

Instructions:

1. Combine the ingredients in a slow cooker.

2. Stir until well combined then cover the slow cooker.

3. Cook on low heat for 7 to 8 hours or on high heat for 4 to 5 hours until the meat is cooked through.

4. Serve the chili hot garnished with diced red onion and shredded cheese.

Baked Chicken Noodle Casserole

Ingredients:

- 2 boneless skinless chicken breasts, chopped

- 1 12-ounce bag egg noodles

- 1 (10 ¾ ounce) can cream of chicken soup

- Skim milk

- 1 large egg, whisked

- 2 cups sliced mushrooms

- 1 ½ cups shredded cheese

Instructions:

1. Preheat the oven to 350°F (175°C).

2. Combine the chicken and noodles in a casserole dish.

3. Pour the soup into a bowl then fill the can with milk and pour it in.

4. Whisk the soup and milk in the egg then stir into the casserole dish with the mushrooms.

5. Cover the dish with foil and bake for 30 to 40 minutes until heated through.

6. Uncover and sprinkle with the cheese.

7. Bake for another 5 minutes or so until the cheese melts.

Cool Ranch Chicken

Ingredients:

- 1 1/4 lb boneless chicken breast

- 1 envelope dry taco mix or alternatively, 2 TBSP homemade

- 1 envelop dry ranch dressing mix or 1 TBSP homemade

- 1 1/2 cups chicken broth

- 1 Cup brown rice

Directions:

1. In a small mixing bowl combine the chicken broth, ranch dressing and taco mix.

2. Add chicken to a slow cooker and cover with chicken broth mixture.

3. Turn the cooker to a low setting and cook covered for 4 to 5 hours.

4. Remove chicken from pot and shred with two forks.

5. Return chicken back to the slow cooker and cook for a further 25 to 30 minutes.

6. Add rice to a pan of boiling water; add a little salt to taste and cook until the rice is soft.

7. Serve with tacos and brown rice.

Day 27:

Breakfast recipes

Bran Muffin

Ingredients

- 6 cups Cereal, all bran
- 2 cups boiling Water
- 4 large Eggs, beaten
- 3 cups Milk, 2%
- 1 cup Olive oil
- 4 cups Wheat flour, whole wheat
- 1 cup Soy flour, stirred
- 3 teaspoons Baking powder
- 5 teaspoons Baking soda
- 1 ½ cups Sugar
- 1 teaspoon Salt

Directions

1. Preheat oven to 400 degree F.

2. In a large bowl, add boiling water to cereal.

3. Let stand for a few minutes.

4. Add eggs, milk and oil. Mix well and set aside.

5. In another bowl, mix flours, baking powder, baking soda, sugar and salt.

6. Mix the two bowls together. Stir well the batter.

Baked Oatmeal

Ingredients

- 2 large Eggs

- 1 cup Milk, fat free

- 1/4 cup Olive oil

- 1/4 cup Applesauce, unsweetened

- 3 cups Oatmeal, instant or quick

- 2 teaspoons Baking powder

- 1/2 cup Splenda, granulated

Directions

1. In a bowl, beat eggs slightly. Add all liquid ingredients together and set aside.

2. Mix oatmeal, baking powder and Splenda.

3. Mix well with egg mixture.

4. Place in greased 9x9 pan. Bake at 350 degrees F for 30 minutes.

Egg Omelet

Ingredients

1. 2 medium Eggs, beaten

2. 1/2 medium Tomato, cut in small chunks

3. 1 medium White mushroom, sliced

Directions

1. Preheat oven to 350 degrees F.

2. Combine eggs, tomato and mushroom.

3. Heat a pan greased with olive oil.

4. Pour egg mixture and bake for 25 minutes or until the center is ready.

Zucchini Bran Muffins

Ingredients

- 3 cups Zucchini, chopped

- 1 cup Carrot, chopped

- 1 ½ cups All-purpose flour

- 1 cup Wheat flour, whole wheat

- 1/2 cup Oat bran, raw

- 1/4 cup Applesauce

- 1 ¼ cups Sugar

- 3/4 cup Canola oil

Directions

1. Preheat oven to 350 degrees F.

2. In a large bowl, mix zucchini, carrot, flours, oat bran, applesauce, sugar and canola oil.

3. Stir well the mixture.

4. Spoon the mixture 2/3 of each muffin pan.

5. Bake for 20-25 minutes and serve.

Lunch Recipes

Fettuccine with Tomatoes and Pesto

Bursting with ripe tomatoes and fresh basil, this dish is the very essence of summer. Keep the heavier tomato sauces for winter, and make this your warm-weather go-to dinner. If you make the pesto in advance, it's a quick and delicious way to have a relaxing dinner after a busy day.

- 1 pound whole-grain fettuccine

- 4 Roma tomatoes, diced

- 2 teaspoons tomato paste

- 1 cup vegetable broth

- 2 garlic cloves, minced

- 1 tablespoon chopped fresh oregano

- 1/2 teaspoon salt

- 1 packed cup fresh basil leaves

- 1/4 cup extra-virgin olive oil

- 1/4 cup grated Parmesan cheese

- 1/4 cup pine nuts

Bring a large stockpot of water to a boil over high heat, and cook the fettuccine according to the package instructions until al dente (still slightly firm). Drain but do not rinse.

Meanwhile, in a large, heavy skillet, combine the tomatoes, tomato paste, broth, garlic, oregano, and salt and stir well. Cook over medium heat for 10 minutes.

In a blender or food processor, combine the basil, olive oil, Parmesan cheese, and pine nuts and blend until smooth.

Stir the pesto into the tomato mixture. Add the pasta and cook, stirring frequently, just until the pasta is well coated and heated through.

Serve immediately.

Dinner Recipes

Bacon-Wrapped Chicken Medallions

Ingredients:

- •1 ½ lbs. boneless skinless chicken breast
- •8 to 10 slices raw bacon
- •½ tsp. paprika
- •½ tsp. chili powder
- •Salt and pepper to taste

Preparation:

1. Preheat your grill to high heat then reduce to medium-high.

2. Cut the chicken breasts into two or three large chunks.

3. Season the chicken with salt and pepper to taste then dust with paprika and chili powder.

4. Wrap each medallion with a slice of bacon then secure it in place with a wooden skewer.

5. Place the skewers on a grill and cook for 3 to 5 minutes on each side until cooked through.

Slow Cooker Beef Stew

Ingredients:

- 4 lbs. boneless bottom round, chopped

- 3 to 4 tablespoons flour

- 2 tablespoons olive oil

- 2 large yellow onions, chopped

- 2 cups chopped carrots

- 4 cups diced Yukon gold potato

- 1 (6-ounce) can tomato paste

- 2 cups beef stock or broth

- 1 cup red wine, dry

- Salt and pepper to taste

Instructions:

1. Heat the oil in a large skillet over medium-high heat.

2. Toss the beef with the flour then add it to the skillet – cook for 2 to 3 minutes until browned.

3. Combine the beef, onions, tomato paste, carrots, and potato in a slow cooker.

4. Stir in the wine and beef broth until well combined then cover the slow cooker.

5. Cook on low heat for 7 to 8 hours or on high heat for 4 hours until the meat is cooked through.

6. Season with salt and pepper to taste and serve hot.

Balsamic Roasted Chicken Legs

Ingredients:

- •2 lbs. raw chicken legs

- •2 tbsp. balsamic vinegar

- •2 tbsp. olive oil

- •1 tsp. onion powder

- •Salt and pepper to taste

Preparation:

1. Preheat the oven to 375°F and lightly grease a glass baking dish.

Day 28:

Breakfast recipes

Fluffy Pancakes

Ingredients

- 1 ½ cups All purpose flour
- 3 ½ teaspoons Baking powder
- 1 large Egg, beaten
- 1 tablespoon Sugar
- 1 ¼ cups Milk, 2%
- 3 tablespoons Butter
- 3/4 teaspoon Salt
- 1 teaspoon Vanilla extract

Directions

1. Preheat oven to 350 degrees F.

2. In a bowl, mix flour, baking powder, egg, sugar, milk, butter, salt and vanilla together.

3. Spoon out to a pan ¼ cup mix per cake.

4. Cook 1-2 minutes or until edges bubble.

5. Flip and cook 1-2 minutes more

6. It's ready to serve.

Baked Oats

Ingredients

- 2 cups Oats

- 6 medium Eggs, beaten

- 1 ¾ cups skim Milk

- 11 ounces dried Fruit, mixed

- 1/2 cup Walnuts, chopped

- 3 tablespoons Coconut oil

- 1 tablespoon Vanilla extract

Directions

1. Soak oats for a few hours.

2. Mix oats, eggs, milk, dried fruit, walnuts, coconut oil and vanilla together.

3. Pour into 9x13 pan and bake at 350 degrees F for 45 minutes.

Cholesterol Free Granola

Ingredients

- 7 packets rolled Oats (1 cup)

- 1 cup Pecans, chopped

- 1 cup Pumpkin seed kernels, raw

- 1 cup Wheat germ

- 1/2 cup ground Flax seed meal

- 3/4 cup Honey

- 1/2 cup Coconut oil, extra virgin

- 1/2 cup Brown sugar

- 2 teaspoons Vanilla extract

Directions

1. Preheat oven to 350 degrees F.

2. Mix oats, pecans, pumpkin seed kernels, wheat germ and flax seed meal in a large bowl.

3. Mix honey, coconut oil, sugar and vanilla in a small saucepan and cook on medium heat until sugar is dissolved.

4. Pour honey mixture over the dry ingredients and mix thoroughly.

5. Place on a flat tray or cookie sheet and bake for 20 minutes.

6. Let it cool completely before storing in an airtight container.

Lunch Recipes

Penne with Roasted Vegetables

Penne has enough heft to hold its own when combined with chunky ingredients. Paired with caramelized roasted veggies, it makes a filling, nutritious meal.

Ingredients:

- 1 large butternut squash, peeled and diced

- 1 large zucchini, diced

- 1 large yellow onion, chopped

- 2 tablespoons extra-virgin olive oil

- 1/2 teaspoon salt

- 1/2 teaspoon freshly ground black pepper

- 1 teaspoon paprika

- 1/2 teaspoon garlic powder

- 1 pound whole-grain penne

- 1/2 cup dry white wine or chicken stock

- 2 tablespoons grated Parmesan cheese

Preparation

Preheat the oven to 400°F. Line a baking sheet with aluminum foil.

In a large bowl, toss the vegetables with the olive oil, then spread them out on the baking sheet. Sprinkle the vegetables with the salt, pepper, paprika, and garlic powder and bake just until fork-tender, 25 to 30 minutes.

Meanwhile, bring a large stockpot of water to a boil over high heat and cook the penne according to the package instructions until al dente (still slightly firm). Drain but do not rinse.

Place 1/2 cup of the roasted vegetables and the wine or stock in a blender or food processor and blend until smooth.

Place the purée in a large skillet and heat over medium-high heat. Add the pasta and cook, stirring, just until heated through.

Serve the pasta and sauce topped with the roasted vegetables. Sprinkle with Parmesan cheese.

Day 29:

Breakfast recipes

Blender Pancakes

Ingredients:

- 1 cup Wheat, whole grains
- 2 tablespoons Sugar
- 1 ½ cups Water
- 2 tablespoons Milk powder
- 1 tablespoon Flax seeds, ground
- 1 dash Salt
- 2 teaspoons Baking powder

Directions

1. Preheat oven to 350 degrees F.

2. In a big bowl, add wheat, sugar and 1 ¼ cups of water and blend for 1 minute.

3. Add milk, flax seeds, ¼ cup of water and salt. Blend for another minute.

4. Add baking powder and blend again.

5. Drop on greased pan in silver dollar-sized pancakes.

6. Flip when bubbles start to form.

Southwestern Chicken Casserole

Ingredients:

- 1 (8-ounce) bag tortilla chips, broken up
- 6 boneless skinless chicken breast, chopped
- 1 cup tomato salsa
- 2 cups shredded Monterey jack cheese

Instructions:

1. Spread the tortilla chips in the bottom of the slow cooker.

2. Place the chicken on top and pour the sauce over it.

3. Sprinkle with cheese then cover the slow cooker.

4. Cook on low heat for 8 hours then serve with sour cream.

Yogurt Pancakes

Ingredients

- 1 cup All-purpose flour

- 1/2 teaspoon Baking soda

- 3/4 teaspoon Baking powder

- 1 large Egg

- 1 1/8 cups Yogurt, fat free

Directions

1. In a bowl, whisk to blend flour, baking soda and baking powder. Set aside.

2. In a separate bowl, mix egg and yogurt until blended.

3. Add dry ingredients and stir until well mixed.

4. Preheat a pan greased with cooking spray.

5. Spread ¼ cup batter on pan into even 4" circle. Flip when browned, around 3 minutes.

6. Bake other side for 2 minutes or until golden.

7. Repeat with the remaining batter.

Stuffed Peppers (Chiles Rellenos)

Ingredients:

- 6 Roasted Poblano Chiles or 12 canned
- 8 ounces queso fresco, cut into thin slices
- 6 large eggs, separated
- ¾ cup flour
- ½ teaspoon salt
- 1 cup canola oil
- 2 cups Roasted Tomatillo Salsa or salsa of your choice

Preparation:

Make a small T-shaped cut at the top of each chile, near the stem.

Cut a slit down the full length of each chile and stuff with a few slices of cheese, dividing the cheese equally. Set aside.

In a large bowl, whisk the egg whites with an electric mixer on high speed until stiff peaks form.

In another bowl, whisk the egg yolks with 1 tablespoon of the flour and the salt.

Gently fold the yolk mixture into the whites, combining until the color is consistent throughout.

In a medium skillet, heat the canola oil over medium-high heat. The oil is ready if it sizzles when you splash a drop of water into it.

Place the remainder of the flour onto a plate.

Carefully dust each chile with the flour and dip each one into the egg batter, coating as evenly as you can.

Place the chiles, open-side down, in the oil and cook until golden brown, about 4 minutes on each side. Place on a platter lined with paper towels to drain.

Repeat until all the chiles are cooked.

In a medium saucepan, warm the salsa until heated through. Remove from the heat, but leave covered on the stove to stay warm.

Place one chile on each plate and pour the salsa over the chiles before serving.

Lunch Recipes

Herb-Roasted Whole Chicken

For a weekend family dinner or a small dinner party, nothing beats the aroma and appeal of a crispy, golden roasted chicken. If there are only one or two of you at home, have this for dinner one night and enjoy the leftovers in salads, sandwiches, or pasta dishes.

Preparation steps:

- 1 (3to 31/2-pound) roasting chicken
- 1 tablespoon extra-virgin olive oil
- 4 rosemary sprigs
- 6 thyme sprigs
- 4 fresh sage leaves
- 1 bay leaf
- 1 teaspoon freshly squeezed lemon juice
- 1 teaspoon salt
- 1/2 teaspoon freshly ground black pepper

Preheat the oven to 400°F. Place a rack inside a large roasting pan.

Rub the olive oil all over the chicken. As you do, gently loosen the skin over the breast to form a pocket.

Slide half of the rosemary and thyme sprigs underneath the skin over the breast, and put the sage leaves, bay leaf, and remaining sprigs inside the cavity.

Rub with the lemon juice and season with salt and pepper.

Roast until an instant-read thermometer inserted into the thigh registers 165°F, 50 to 60 minutes. Remove from the oven and allow to rest for 10 minutes before carving.

Oven-Poached Cod

Cod is a firm, mild fish that is a terrific source of omega-3 fats. It cooks up easily, takes on the flavors of other ingredients readily, and isn't too expensive, so it's particularly suited to seafood novices. If you have an oven-safe skillet, this is a one-pan meal that makes for easy cleanup.

- 4 (6-ounce) cod filets

- 1/2 teaspoon salt

- 1/2 teaspoon freshly ground black pepper

- 1/2 cup dry white wine

- 1/2 cup seafood or vegetable stock

- 2 garlic cloves, minced

- 1 bay leaf

- 1 teaspoon chopped fresh sage

- 4 rosemary sprigs for garnish

Preheat the oven to 375°F.

Season each filet with salt and pepper and place in a large ovenproof skillet or baking pan. Add the wine, stock, garlic, bay leaf, and sage and cover. Bake until the fish flakes easily with a fork, about 20 minutes.

Use a spatula to remove the filet from the skillet. Place the poaching liquid over high heat and cook, stirring frequently, until reduced by half, about 10 minutes. (Do this in a small saucepan if you used a baking pan.)

To serve, place a filet on each plate and drizzle with the reduced poaching liquid.

Garnish each with a fresh rosemary sprig.

Serves 4.

Dinner Recipes

Cheesy Ranch Potatoes

Ingredients

- 2 lb small red potatoes

- 1 (8 oz) package cream cheese, softened

- 1 (10 3/4 oz) can cream of potato soup

- 1 envelope ranch salad dressing mix

- 1 c. shredded cheddar cheese

Instructions

1. Clean the potatoes and cut into quarters

2. Using a large mixing bowl combine the soup, salad dressing and cream cheese then stir in the shredded cheese.

3. Add the potatoes to a slow cooker and pour the cream cheese mixture over potatoes.

4. Set the slow cooker on the low cover and cook for 7 to 8 hours until the potatoes are soft.

Day 30:

Breakfast recipes

Flour Tortillas

Ingredients:

- 2 cups flour

- 1 teaspoon salt

- 1 teaspoon baking soda

- 1 tablespoon lard or margarine

- ½ cup cold water

Preparation steps:

1. Preheat oven to 350°.

2. Mix together all the ingredients well. If the dough sticks to your hands, add more flour, 1 teaspoon at a time, until it doesn't stick.

3. Divide the dough and roll into balls about the size of golf balls.

4. Flatten the balls between 2 sheets of wax paper. If they stick, scrape them off, add more flour, and start over. Flatten to about ¼-inch thick.

5. Place the tortillas on an ungreased baking sheet and bake in the oven for about 2 minutes. Flip and bake for 2 more minutes, or until lightly browned.

Muffins with coconut Nutella

Ingredients

- 350 gr of flour 00

- 200 grams of sugar

- 2 teaspoons of baking powder

- 2 eggs

- 250ml of milk

- 80g of butter

- 50g of plain yogurt

- 120 g of coconut flour

Preparation steps

1. In two spacious bowls you place the flour in the center of the yeast and sugar.

2. In two other bowls, beat the eggs with the milk and melted butter warmed.

3. Add the liquid to the dry compound, as is usually done to prepare the muffins, stir and mix well.

4. Add the coconut flour and yogurt in large bowl

5. Mix until it forms a smooth and homogeneous.

6. Place paper baking cups in the aluminum (instead of the buttered and floured muffin tins) and pour two teaspoons of coconut compound alternating with 1 tablespoon of the mixture with Nutella, then again two coconut and one with Nutella, and so on until reaching the edge of the paper cups of paper.

7. Arrange all the cups with coconut and chocolate muffins on a baking sheet.

8. Bake the muffins with coconut and Nutella at 180 ° C in a preheated oven and cook for 20 minutes.

9. Let the muffins cool in the coconut and Nutella, then remove them from the molds and serve.

Custar Donuts

Ingredients

- 2 egg yolks

- 2 tablespoons of sugar

- 2 tablespoons of flour

- 200 ml of milk

- 1 tablespoon of vanilla essence

- Powdered sugar

Preparation Steps:

1. Dissolving the yeast in the lukewarm milk, add 100 grams of flour and mix.

2. Cover the bowl with plastic wrap and let rise for 30 minutes.

3. In a large bowl place 150 grams of flour and lemon peel and pour in the center.

4. Begin to work the mixture gradually incorporating the flour.

5. Beat the egg yolks with the sugar then add the melted butter and warmed vanilla essence.

6. Add the egg mixture to the dough and keep working until you get a smooth and soft dough adding the other 50 grams of flour if the dough is sticky trope.

7. Put the dough in a bowl for 2 hours by covering with plastic.

8. Prepare the custard by mixing the yolks with the sugar, add the flour and stir.

Add the milk little by little and a tablespoon of vanilla extract and put the mixture on the stove.

Lunch Recipes

Dilly Baked Salmon

Salmon paired with dill is a culinary classic, and it's especially delicious prepared with a touch of citrus and a little olive oil. Baking fish in foil packets maximizes flavor and minimizes mess.

Ingredients:

- 4 (6-ounce) salmon filets

- 2 tablespoons extra-virgin olive oil

- 1/2 teaspoon salt

- 1/4 teaspoon freshly ground black pepper

- Juice of large Valencia orange or tangerine

- 4 teaspoons orange or tangerine zest

- 4 tablespoons chopped fresh dill

Preparation

Preheat the oven to 375°F. Prepare four 10-inch-long pieces of aluminum foil.

Rub each salmon filet on both sides with the olive oil. Season each with salt and pepper and place one in the center of each piece of foil.

Drizzle the orange juice over each piece of fish and top with 1 teaspoon orange zest and 1 tablespoon dill.

Flank Steak Spinach Salad

Flank steak is an especially lean cut, which makes it a top choice for those occasional meals when you'd like to serve red meat. Incorporating it into a salad makes the meat, and your grocery dollar, go a lot farther.

- 1 pound flank steak

- 1 teaspoon extra-virgin olive oil

- 1 tablespoon garlic powder

- 1/2 teaspoon salt

- 1/2 teaspoon freshly ground black pepper

- 4 cups baby spinach leaves

- 10 cherry tomatoes, halved

- 10 cremini or white mushrooms, sliced

- 1 small red onion, thinly sliced

- 1/2 red bell pepper, thinly sliced

Preheat the broiler. Line a baking sheet with aluminum foil.

Rub the top of the flank steak with the olive oil, garlic powder, salt, and pepper and let sit for 10 minutes before placing under the broiler. Broil for 5 minutes on each side for medium rare. Allow the meat to rest on a cutting board for 10 minutes.

Meanwhile, in a large bowl, combine the spinach, tomatoes, mushrooms, onion, and bell pepper and toss well.

To serve, divide the salad among 4 dinner plates. Slice the steak on the diagonal and place 4 to 5 slices on top of each salad. Serve with your favorite vinaigrette.

Serves 4.

Dinner Recipes

Bacon-Wrapped Chicken Medallions

Ingredients:

- 1 ½ lbs. boneless skinless chicken breast

- 8 to 10 slices raw bacon

- ½ tsp. paprika

- ½ tsp. chili powder

- Salt and pepper to taste

Preparation:

1. Preheat your grill to high heat then reduce to medium-high.

2. Cut the chicken breasts into two or three large chunks.

3. Season the chicken with salt and pepper to taste then dust with paprika and chili powder.

4. Wrap each medallion using a bacon slice then secure it in place with a wooden skewer.

5. Place the skewers on a grill and cook for 3 to 5 minutes on each side until cooked through.

Orange Grilled Chicken with Mango Salsa

Ingredients:

- •4 boneless skinless chicken breast
- •2 tbsp. fresh orange juice
- •1 tbsp. olive oil
- •Salt and pepper to taste
- •1 ripe mango, pitted and diced
- •1 small tomato, diced
- •½ cup seedless cucumber diced small
- •¼ cup fresh chopped cilantro

Preparation:

1. Heat your grill to high heat then reduce to medium-high.

2. Whisk together the orange juice and olive oil in a small bowl.

3. Season the chicken with salt and pepper to taste then brush with the marinade.

4. Place the chicken breasts on the grill and cook for 10 minutes.

5. Turn the chicken and brush again with marinade.

6. Cook the chicken for another 8 to 10 minutes until it is cooked through.

7. Combine the remaining ingredients in a bowl and serve over the hot chicken.

Hungarian Goulash

Ingredients

- 2 pounds stew meat, cut in 1" cubes

- 1 large onion, sliced

- 1 clove garlic, minced

- 1/2 cup ketchup

- 2 tablespoons Worcestershire sauce

- 1 tablespoon brown sugar

- 2 teaspoons salt

- 2 teaspoons paprika

- 1/2 teaspoon dry mustard

- 1 cup water

- 1/2 cup flour

Instructions

1. Add the diced stewing meat to a slow cooker and cover with the sliced onions.

2. In a large bowl mix together the mustard, paprika, salt, sugar, Worcestershire sauce,

ketchup, and garlic. Mix with the water and pour over the meat.

3. Set your slow cooker on a low setting and cook for 8 to 9 hours.

4. 15 minutes before serving turn the cooker setting to high.

5. Add the flour to a small amount of water and mix thoroughly, add to meat mixture and stir.

6. Leave to thicken for 10 to 15 minutes.

7. Serve with hot white rice.

Conclusion

The human mind is unveiling the hidden realities confined within the internal and external systems of human body. The research and intellectual efforts of the human race have uncovered a lot of hidden realities present in the surrounding. Same is the case of knowing details about the internal system of human body and mind. The overall healthy human body is governed by a number of connected and intermingled factors, which pertain to both physical and psychological factors. It is because of this deeper knowledge that we are better able to address the issues of modern-day human beings. Deeper understanding has led us to entertain the unattended corners of human life.

When it comes to overall body wellness and outlook, one of the most reported issues for modern-day population is the increasingly high rate of obesity. Almost all sorts of efforts are put forward to overcome obesity but it has entered after a change in the overall eating habits as well as in the living standards of modern men. So fighting for it is not easy.

Well, it doesn't involve any sort of magic; in fact, it is purely based up science. Scientists do believe that the difference between the effect of placebo and green tea on the metabolic system's essentially caused by the antioxidants found in the green tea, which have the natural competence to enhance the rate of metabolism. These particular antioxidants are known as the catechins.

Spice Things Up: A study has unearthed an interesting fact that the intake of hot peppers could boost the basal metabolism of an individual. The basal metabolism is basically the amount of calories which are burned by the body when it is at rest. One of the biggest reasons behind the metabolism enhancing property of hot pepper is a compound which is known as capsaicin. Capsaicin is naturally found in cayenne peppers and jalapeno, which could enhance the stress hormones which are released by the human body like adrenaline, eventually which can accelerate the metabolic system and a person's competence to incinerate calories.

Additionally, consuming hot peppers can also reduce the appetite. Therefore, it is good to spice up the stir fried vegetables and eat salsa or chilies with low calories.

One could eat them by putting on the baked potatoes or salads. This is definitely a one good way to shed off the pounds in a faster and safe way without spending hours in the gym or taking unhealthful weight loss supplements.

www.ingramcontent.com/pod-product-compliance
Lightning Source LLC
Chambersburg PA
CBHW060249290526
45789CB00001B/251